Regional Anesthesia in Trauma: A Case-Based Approach

Regional Anesthesia in Trauma: A Case-Based Approach

Jeff Gadsden MD, FRCPC, FANZCA
Regional Anesthesia, St. Luke's-Roosevelt Hospital Center and Clinical Anesthesiology, Columbia University College of Physicians and Surgeons, New York, USA

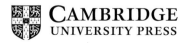

CAMBRIDGE UNIVERSITY PRESS
Cambridge, New York, Melbourne, Madrid, Cape Town,
Singapore, São Paulo, Delhi, Mexico City

Cambridge University Press
The Edinburgh Building, Cambridge CB2 8RU, UK

Published in the United States of America by
Cambridge University Press, New York

www.cambridge.org
Information on this title: www.cambridge.org/9781107602236

First published 2012

Printed in the United States of America by Edwards Brothers

A catalogue record for this publication is available from the British Library

Library of Congress Cataloging in Publication data
Gadsden, Jeff, 1972–
Regional anesthesia in trauma : a case-based approach / Jeff Gadsden.
    p.   ;   cm.
Includes bibliographical references and index.
ISBN 978-1-107-60223-6 (pbk.)
I. Title.
[DNLM: 1. Anesthesia, Conduction – methods.   2. Pain
Management – methods.   3.   Wounds and Injuries – surgery.   WO 300]
617.9′64–dc23

                                                                2012020246

ISBN 978-1-107-60223-6 Paperback

Matthews
Medical Books

Gadsden, Jeff MD
Columbia Univ
Regional Anesthesia in Trauma

ED# 01 PAGES: 141 Softcover

Cambridge, UK Cambridge Univers, C2012
9781107602236

DATE					
01/16/13					
LIST PRICE					
55.00		GENERAL SUBJECT		COPIES	FUND
DISCOUNT					
17.00%	LC CLASS			1	
NET PRICE					
45.65					
NLM CLASS					
WO 300	RD84	Surgery			

Contents

Preface

Trauma is associated with a substantial burden of pain that can be challenging to manage, especially in the face of other priorities such as resuscitation and the diagnosis of multi-system injuries. Complicating this is the fact that traditional analgesics, such as opioids or non-steroidal anti-inflammatory drugs, may be contraindicated or potentially harmful in this population, especially in those with head or chest injuries. Under-treated pain resulting from trauma can be disabling and has been found to lead to both chronic pain and psychological distress long after the injury heals. These factors, in part, have fueled the demand for the increased use of regional analgesic techniques in the setting of trauma. What used to be an uncommon analgesic modality has become much more widespread, particularly since the advent of ultrasound guidance, which has largely demystified nerve blocks for many and made them part of everyday practice in the operating room, the emergency department, the intensive care unit, and in the battlefield.

This book is organized into two sections: the first three chapters serve as an introduction to the concept of pain management during trauma and the importance of high-quality pain control in injured patients; the remaining 18 chapters are case-based discussions, each starting with a clinical vignette and followed by question and answer-style examination of the relevant issues. Throughout the course of the case chapters, principal regional anesthetic and analgesic techniques are fully described with the aid of ultrasound images. However, more than just a how-to book, the theoretical and often controversial issues that inform the clinical decision making are explored, so that the reader gains a thorough understanding of the landscape of regional anesthetic practice in trauma care.

Although regional anesthesia is traditionally the domain of anesthesiologists, this book has been written for a broader audience, recognizing that acute care clinicians of many varieties such as emergency medicine physicians, intensivists, military medics, and others may benefit from an examination of these issues. It is my hope that the lives of injured might be improved by an increased awareness and utilization of the techniques described in this book.

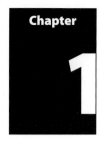

Chapter

1

Principles of pain management in trauma care

Introduction

Pain management in the trauma setting can be very challenging. There are multiple barriers to effective analgesia for trauma patients, such as the overwhelming priority of resuscitation and treatment of life- and limb-threatening injuries, fear of causing harm owing to side effects and an underestimation of a high level of pain intensity. Trauma patients are frequently unable to communicate because of the need for sedation, mechanical ventilation, etc., which can impair adequate pain assessment. Untreated pain in the injured patient is not merely a nuisance, but can increase patient fear and anxiety and have a detrimental effect on physiologic parameters, leading to significant delays in long-term physical and emotional recovery. Traumatologists are becoming better at recognizing the adverse outcomes associated with uncontrolled pain, as well as at implementing pain control solutions that are well matched to each specific patient's need.

The importance of pain management in trauma care

Acute pain represents a physical and emotional burden that can linger for long after the inciting injury heals. It is well described that under-treated acute pain can lead to the development of chronic pain syndromes (see Chapter 3), and this is as true for the trauma patient as it is for the surgical patient undergoing mastectomy or thoracotomy. Certain pain syndromes, such as complex regional pain syndrome (CRPS), are unique to trauma, and the severity and duration may be influenced with the proper and early use of pain management techniques. Inadequate analgesia has been associated with thromboembolic events, pulmonary complications, and increased ICU and hospital length of stay. Post-traumatic stress disorder (PTSD) is an affliction characterized by intrusive thoughts, nightmares and flashbacks of a past traumatic event, avoidance of reminders of trauma, hypervigilance, anxiety and sleep disturbance, all of which lead to considerable social, occupational and interpersonal dysfunction. Above all else, continued pain represents needless suffering, for which there is no valid excuse. Trauma care providers of all types (prehospital emergency medical technicians (EMTs) and paramedics, nurses and physicians) should make the evaluation and prompt, safe treatment of pain one of their prime directives.

Changing patterns of analgesia

The most common approach to pain management in trauma patients is intravenous opioids. This is true in the prehospital setting, where paramedics and EMTs administer opioids (typically morphine) for acute pain related to injuries or medical pain; it is also true in the emergency room as well as through the perioperative period. Opioids are excellent analgesics, work quickly and are a rational choice when patients have multiple injuries. However, opioids have a wide variety of side effects that can impact patient physiology and disposition, including:

- Respiratory depression
- Nausea and vomiting
- Pruritus
- Constipation
- Vasodilation and hypotension (especially in hypovolemia)
- Immunosuppression
- Increased staffing requirement to monitor patient
- Increased length of stay in emergency department or recovery room.

Anesthesiologists have long been strong advocates for the use of multimodal analgesia in surgical patients. Its use is also well suited to the acute trauma setting, where it leads to a reduction in opioid requirements and opioid-related side effects. Common multimodal agents used in the care of trauma patients are listed in Table 1.1. While there are a multitude

Table 1.1 Parenteral multimodal agents commonly used in the trauma setting

Agent	IV/IM Dosage	Notes
Acetaminophen (paracetamol)	1 g IV/PO q 4–6 hours to a maximum of 4 g/day	Very safe profile, even in cases with traumatic liver laceration Hepatotoxicity in very large doses No antiplatelet effect
Ketorolac	30 mg, then 15–30 mg every 6 hours	↓Bone fusion if used in large doses/ prolonged duration Gastric irritation, platelet inhibition Caution with renal insufficiency and asthma
Ketamine	250 mcg/kg loading dose, then 5–10 mcg/kg/h infusion	Potent analgesic ↑Secretions Hallucinations (more with racemic, less with S-enantiomer) ↑Intracranial pressure ↑Sympathetic activity (bronchodilation, ↑HR/ BP): good for hypotensive/hypovolemic patient
Alpha-2 agonists	Clonidine Dexmedetomidine (bolus 1 mcg/kg, followed by infusion of 0.3–0.4 mcg/kg/h)	Sedation Hypotension Bradycardia
Entonox	Inhaled 50:50 mixture of nitrous oxide and oxygen	Moderate analgesic Nausea/vomiting Contraindicated in head injury, pneumothorax

of available analgesics, for practical purposes only parenteral medications have been included, as the enteral route is often unavailable in these patients.

Regional anesthesia, particularly the use of peripheral nerve blocks, has been growing in popularity for the treatment of the acutely injured patient, both in civilian and in military medical systems. Its myriad advantages in this setting include:

- Reduction in sedative medications (especially important in avoiding respiratory depression or neurologic impairment in those with chest or head injuries)
- Reduction in other opioid-related side effects such as nausea, vomiting, pruritis, constipation and urinary retention
- Decreased risk of hypotension compared to some conscious sedation techniques, especially if the patient is hypovolemic
- Intense analgesia targeted at the injured area and nowhere else
- Decreased length of stay in the emergency room and recovery room
- Attenuated stress response to injury
- Improved safety and comfort of transport
- Decreased need for medical supervision, staffing
- Possible reduction in chronic pain syndromes and PTSD
- Decreased costs compared with conscious sedation techniques for procedural analgesia.

Not every patient is suitable for regional anesthesia techniques; similarly, the provision of regional anesthesia requires specialized training as well as a thorough understanding of the risks and benefits of performing blocks, which include nerve injury, local anesthetic systemic toxicity and inadvertent puncture of neighboring structures. Different techniques may be better suited for different phases of the patient's recovery phase – for example, a single patient might receive a femoral block in the field, intercostal blocks in the emergency department, an epidural in the operating room and a continuous paravertebral catheter in the ICU, all within a period of several days.

The widespread use of ultrasonography for diagnosis of intra-abdominal and intra-thoracic injuries makes the traumatologist, whether surgeon, anesthesiologist or emergency medicine specialist, well positioned to become facile at ultrasound-guided nerve blocks. There have been an increasing number of trials showing that ultrasound improves block success and is faster than traditional nerve stimulator or landmark methods; in addition, the incidence of inadvertent vascular puncture is decreased, just as it is when using ultrasound for jugular vein cannulation. Ultrasound is rapidly becoming, if not a standard of care, a technology that few experienced regional anesthesiologists wish to do without. For that reason, most of the techniques described in this book are of the ultrasound-guided variety, with a few exceptions.

Further reading

Fosnocht, D. E., Swanson, E. R., Barton, E. D. (2005). Changing attitudes about pain and pain control in emergency medicine. *Emergency Medicine Clinics of North America*, **23**, 297–306.

Gadsden, J., Todd, K. (2006). Regional anesthesia and acute pain management in the emergency department. In: Hadzic, A. (ed.) *Textbook of Regional Anesthesia and Acute Pain Management*, 1st edn. New York: McGraw-Hill Professional, pp. 955–66.

Grabinsky, A., Sharar, S. R. (2009). Regional anesthesia for acute traumatic injuries in the emergency room. *Expert Review of Neurotherapeutics*, **9**, 1677–90.

Malchow, R. J., Black, I. H. (2008). The evolution of pain management in the critically ill trauma patient: Emerging concepts from the global war on terrorism. *Critical Care Medicine*, **36**, S346–57.

Todd, K. H., Ducharme, J., Choiniere, M. *et al.* (2007). Pain in the emergency department: results of the pain and emergency medicine initiative (PEMI) multicenter study. *The Journal of Pain: Official Journal of the American Pain Society*, **8**, 460–6.

Wu, J. J., Lollo, L., Grabinsky, A. (2011). Regional anesthesia in trauma medicine. *Anesthesiology Research and Practice*, **2011**, 713281.

Chapter 2

Acute pain, regional anesthesia and the stress response

Introduction

Trauma to the body, whether surgical or accidental, results in a barrage of noxious afferent input to the central nervous system (CNS). This in turn triggers a cascade of endocrine, metabolic and inflammatory events that, taken together, are known as the "stress response." The stress response is an adaptive physiologic process that aids in survival by providing fuel substrates (in the form of glucose, amino acids and fatty acids), circulatory support (by promoting the renal retention of water and by the release of catecholamines) and a hypercoagulable state. In the short term, this strategy is probably protective during "fight or flight" situations, but in a medical setting, this response, if untreated, is accompanied by undesirable physiologic effects that lead to increased morbidity following trauma. This chapter will discuss the stress response and the role that regional anesthesia may play in attenuating its effects.

Metabolic response

Glucose levels are elevated following trauma, and are directly proportional to the degree of tissue injury. This is the result of the secretion of counter-regulatory hormones such as cortisol and glucagon which promote increased glucose production (gluconeogenesis and glycogenolysis), decreased glucose utilization, enhanced renal absorption of filtered glucose and resistance to insulin. Under conditions of stress, membrane proteins are expressed that allow this excessive glucose to enter cells in the endothelium, brain and liver. Intracellular glucose glycosylates proteins (e.g. immunoglobulins), rendering them ineffective. Several studies have demonstrated a direct relationship between in-hospital glucose levels and mortality, highlighting the need for strict control of this metabolic derangement.

Accelerated protein catabolism and release of amino acids occurs at the same time during stress. This can lead to a significant loss in lean muscle mass, impaired wound healing and compromised immune function. Net protein loss can exceed 200 g of nitrogen (approximately 6 kg of lean tissue) following trauma. Hepatic protein synthesis is prioritized to generate acute phase proteins such as C-reactive protein at the expense of constitutive proteins such as albumin.

Free fatty acids are released during stress owing to sympathetically mediated lipolysis. Elevated free fatty acids are a cardiovascular risk factor, having been demonstrated to depress myocardial contractility, increase myocardial oxygen consumption and to impair endothelium-dependent vasodilation.

Table 2.1 Hormonal response to stress

Hormone	Change with trauma	Effect
Adrenocorticotropic hormone (ACTH)	↑	Release of cortisol from adrenal cortex
Growth hormone	↑	Insulin resistance, lipolysis
Antidiuretic hormone	↑	Retention of free water by kidney
Cortisol	↑	Glucose production, protein catabolism, lipolysis, anti-inflammatory
Aldosterone	↑	Sodium and water retention
Insulin	↓	Hyperglycemia
Glucagon	↑	Gluconeogenesis

These metabolic changes can be seen as a redistribution of macronutrients from reserve tissue (skeletal muscle and fat) to more active tissues (liver and bone marrow) for reasons of host defense and visceral protein synthesis (Table 2.1).

Autonomic response

Immediately following traumatic injury, the sympathetic nervous system is activated, causing an increase in plasma levels of epinephrine and norepinephrine. This leads to an increase in heart rate, contractility, arterial blood pressure, left ventricular stroke work and the incidence of arrhythmias.

Regional anesthesia and the stress response

Since the nervous system is the catalyst for initiating the stress response, it seems to be a logical target for mitigating the physiologic derangements seen with trauma. In particular, blocking the afferent nociceptive traffic from entering the CNS prevents activation of the hypothalamic–pituitary axis and the subsequent release of adrenocorticotropic hormone (ACTH), growth hormone and antidiuretic hormone.

Of the different regional techniques, epidural blockade has been the most extensively studied. Most well-performed studies have been carried out in elective surgery and appear to agree that extensive epidural blockade that "matches" the dermatomal distribution of the incision can be effective at ameliorating the neuroendocrine response, provided that it is initiated before surgery and maintained for at least 48–72 hours postoperatively. For example, during hysterectomy, epidural blockade of levels T4 to S5 for hysterectomy effectively negated any increase in cortisol or glucose. This is more difficult to achieve with upper abdominal or thoracic surgical procedures – in a study with blocks up to C6, glycemic changes were shown to be inhibited but the rise in cortisol was not. The reasons for this are not clear, but may have to do with inadequate sympathetic blockade and the continued release of ACTH from the pituitary.

Studies investigating the role of peripheral nerve blocks in attenuating the surgical stress response have shown mixed results. These techniques appear to be effective at attenuating the response during cataract surgery under retrobulbar block, and for thoracic surgery using paravertebral blockade. On the other hand, knee arthroplasty patients continued to experience a rise in neuroendocrine hormone levels during total knee arthroplasty using femoral and sciatic blockade. An explanation for this is that the continued neural input from the obturator and/or lateral femoral cutaneous nerves activates the hormonal cascade despite the blockade of most of the neural input.

Regional anesthetic techniques have been shown to confer beneficial effects on multiple organ systems, probably in large part because of the ability of neural blockade to control the stress response. These include reductions in pulmonary complications, deep venous thromboses, pulmonary emboli and myocardial infarction.

For the traumatically injured patient, the opportunity to place a regional block in advance of the insult is clearly lost. However, theoretically there appears to be a benefit from the abolition of the *continued* nociceptive barrage. The nature and timing of such a reduction has not yet been fully characterized. In the meantime, regional blocks in trauma patients have not been shown to be inferior in this regard and have multiple other benefits to recommend them, including superior analgesia, improved rehabilitation and the ability to avoid opioids and opioid-related side effects.

Further reading

Blackburn, G. L. (2011). Metabolic considerations in management of surgical patients. *The Surgical Clinics of North America*, **91**, 467–80.

Brøchner, A. C., Toft, P. (2009). Pathophysiology of the systemic inflammatory response after major accidental trauma. *Scandinavian Journal of Trauma, Resuscitation and Emergency Medicine*, **17**, 43.

Bromage, P. R., Shibata, H. R., Willoughby, H. W. (1971). Influence of prolonged epidural blockade on blood sugar and cortisol responses to operations upon the upper part of the abdomen and the thorax. *Surgery, Gynecology & Obstetrics*, **132**, 1051–6.

Desborough, J. P. (2000). The stress response to trauma and surgery. *British Journal of Anaesthesia*, **85**, 109–17.

Rodgers, A., Walker, N., Schug, S. *et al.* (2000). Reduction of postoperative mortality and morbidity with epidural or spinal anaesthesia: results from overview of randomised trials. *BMJ*, **321**, 1493.

Chapter 3

The progression from acute to chronic pain

Introduction

Acute pain is an adaptive response that is protective and serves to minimize further injury. During the process of recovery from the inciting event, a steady stream of nociceptive input is received by the spinal cord and transmitted to the higher centers in the CNS. This is prolonged by the sensitization of peripheral nerve endings to non-noxious stimulation by inflammatory mediators released as a result of the injury (peripheral sensitization). Over time, this afferent barrage causes hyperexcitation of central neurons and a decrease in the threshold required to cause a painful stimulus (central sensitization). If allowed to continue unabated, this sensitization can result in a chronic pain condition, where the original injury has healed, but the pain is maintained by the abnormally functioning nerves themselves (neuropathic pain). It is estimated that over 20% of adults in the western world experience chronic pain during their lifetime, accounting for a tremendous burden of suffering and cost to healthcare systems. Chronic pain is often defined as pain lasting greater than 3–6 months after the initial injury.

Chronic post-trauma pain

The incidence of chronic pain following severe trauma is dependent on several factors, such as the type of injury and psychological health. One study of 90 individuals that suffered severe trauma found that 44% reported accident-related pain 3 years after the accident. Those with chronic pain showed significantly more symptoms of PTSD, depression and anxiety, more disability and more days off work.

Common causes of post-traumatic pain syndromes include headache following traumatic brain injury, CRPS following injury to (usually) a distal extremity, post-traumatic abdominal pain and pain related to spinal injury (bony vertebral or spinal cord injury).

Patients suffering traumatic amputations have very specific patterns of chronic pain, including residual limb pain (stump pain), phantom limb sensation (any sensation in the missing limb except pain) and phantom limb pain. This last entity is present in up to 50–80% of amputees, and may be severe enough to interfere with a patient's work and social life. One of the factors that seems to be related to a higher risk of developing phantom limb pain is poor control of preoperative pain. In one randomized controlled study of 65 patients undergoing amputation, quality analgesia with either epidural or intravenous opioids for 48 hours prior to and 48 hours following surgery led to decreased incidence and intensity of phantom limb pain at 6 months.

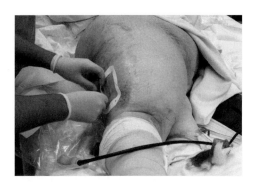

Figure 3.1 Popliteal sciatic catheter being placed prior to an amputation revision.

"Pre-emptive" versus "preventive" analgesia

The idea that providing analgesia in advance of a painful stimulus might reduce pain intensity afterwards is not new. In the early 1990s the concept of "pre-emptive" analgesia was proposed; this held that a treatment initiated before a painful stimulus will prevent or reduce subsequent pain compared to an identical treatment administered after the stimulus. An example is a nerve block administered for hand surgery – when performed before the operation, the CNS does not receive the barrage of afferent input (until the block wears off); if the same block is put in *postoperatively* following a general anesthetic, the spinal cord immediately begins to receive nociceptive input and is likely to begin the process of central sensitization. Note that in this particular example, while central sensitization is (temporarily) suspended, peripheral sensitization is still occurring.

Preventive analgesia, in contrast, is based on the principle that the only way to guarantee the prevention of central sensitization (and therefore CNS neuroplastic changes that lead to chronic pain) is to maintain the analgesic treatment for the duration of the inflammatory stimulus. In the above example, this might mean placing a peripheral nerve catheter rather than performing a single injection block, and maintaining a local anesthetic infusion for days, and possibly weeks, depending on the nature of the stimulus.

The data supporting the existence of pre-emptive analgesia are limited. This is not surprising when the intensity of post-injury neural input is considered in relation to a brief delay in central sensitization. While the idea of preventive analgesia is an attractive one, a similar lack of evidence prevents strong recommendations of any kind regarding its efficacy. Notwithstanding, the provision of prolonged analgesia surrounding a surgical insult is not only theoretically appealing for any possible role in prevention of chronic pain, but it is also good medicine, as the relief of suffering is one of our primary goals.

Chronic pain and regional anesthesia

Various modalities have been employed in an attempt to invoke preventive analgesia. These include various antihyperalgesic medications such as ketamine, gabapentinoids, antidepressants and anti-inflammatory drugs. While some reports show promising results, these are primarily drugs that have shown utility for neuropathic pain of other origin (i.e. postherpetic neuralgia, diabetic neuropathy, etc.). As such, it is difficult to expect these relatively mild therapies to have an effect on an acute pain process that is severe, unrelenting and can last weeks following the moment of injury.

Although the ultimate solution to this problem will likely involve multimodal therapy, many anesthesiologists feel that continuous neural blockade is the closest thing possible to a preventive "magic bullet." In the trauma setting, it can be initiated as close to the time of injury as is practical, and maintained throughout the period of convalescence. Much of the evidence for safety and tolerability of long-term perineural catheter techniques has come following the military experience in Iraq and Afghanistan. Several authors have reported large series of wounded soldiers who have been instrumented with peripheral catheters and portable infusion pumps, then transported thousands of miles to regional medical centers or definitive care hospitals in their home country in comfort and safety (see Chapter 9). The safety record for these catheters, some of which have remained in place for weeks, is excellent, with low complication rates. What remains to be seen is the effect that these prolonged interventions will have on the incidence of chronic pain in this population. The vast majority of these patients have suffered extremity injury, and many are amputees. As the global war on terror continues, we are certain to accumulate evidence on this topic that will be of use to providers of acute pain services in the civilian arena.

Further reading

Dahl, J. B., Kehlet, H. (2011). Preventive analgesia. *Current Opinion in Anaesthesiology*, **24**, 331–8.

Jenewein, J., Moergeli, H., Wittmann, L. *et al.* (2009). Development of chronic pain following severe accidental injury. Results of a 3-year follow-up study. *Journal of Psychosomatic Research*, **66**, 119–26.

Karanikolas, M., Aretha, D., Tsolakis, I. *et al.* (2011). Optimized perioperative analgesia reduces chronic phantom limb pain

intensity, prevalence, and frequency: a prospective, randomized, clinical trial. *Anesthesiology*, **114**, 1144–54.

Lavand'homme, P. (2011). The progression from acute to chronic pain. *Current Opinion in Anaesthesiology*, **24**, 545–50.

McGreevy, K., Bottros, M. M., Raja, S. N. (2011). Preventing chronic pain following acute pain: risk factors, preventive strategies, and their efficacy. *European Journal of Pain Supplements*, **5**, 365–72.

Prehospital regional anesthesia

Key aspects of case

1. Role of regional anesthesia for trauma in the prehospital setting.
2. Fat embolism syndrome.

Case presentation

A 34-year-old female is making a turn in her car when she is struck on the driver's side by another vehicle at moderate speed (65 km/h). The emergency medical services (EMS) team arrives within 7 minutes and includes two paramedics and a physician. The crew finds the woman sitting up in the driver's seat, awake and responsive, with a Glasgow Coma Score (GCS) of 15. She is maintaining her own airway and breath sounds are equal bilaterally. Vitals are BP 139/92, HR 113, RR 23. Her face and scalp are bloody owing to multiple lacerations from flying glass, and she is complaining of severe pain localized to her right thigh. Following spinal immobilization, she is extricated from the vehicle. A quick survey reveals what appears to be a right femoral fracture based on her pain and the obvious deformity. There are no other obvious serious injuries.

Case discussion

Describe the concepts of "scoop and run" and "stay and play" as they relate to prehospital care of trauma patients

In trauma care, prehospital priorities generally include management of the compromised airway, control of ongoing external bleeding, immobilization of the spine if indicated, and, in cases of low blood pressure from presumed hemorrhage, initiation of intravenous fluid resuscitation.

The phrase "scoop and run" refers to the expeditious evacuation of patients by the EMS team to a trauma facility where definitive care can be implemented, without delay for involved on-scene advanced life support therapy. Supporters of this school of thought cite evidence that prolonged attempts at endotracheal intubation, vascular access and stabilization of a patient at the scene serve to delay proper care at the hospital, and may in fact increase morbidity and mortality.

The concept of "stay and play" is based on the idea that provision of initial resuscitation and management at the scene permits the transfer of a more stable patient to hospital. Proponents of this strategy state that the extra time spent promptly treating major injuries at the scene is preferable to transporting a patient who continues to suffer the ongoing deleterious effects of their injuries. Studies also exist demonstrating improved outcomes using this method.

This is clearly a controversial topic, and several factors determine which strategy is advantageous. First and foremost is the degree of training of the EMS team. In many parts of the world, including many European nations, EMS teams are staffed by physicians (often anesthesiologists or intensivists) highly trained in resuscitative and trauma medicine. These tend to be the systems that benefit most from on-scene triaging, evaluation and therapeutic intervention, as complex medical decision-making and management can take place without the need for communication with a remote physician. Conversely, some systems (such as the USA) employ paramedics, EMTs or firefighters as first responders. In these systems, there is a limited set of interventions that can be performed in the field, and decision-making capability is more restricted; it may be more appropriate in these cases to focus on expeditious transfer.

Transfer time to hospital is also a factor. In rural areas where time to hospital might be upwards of an hour, there is more rationale for spending time at the scene tending to major injuries. On the other hand, in urban environments, where transfer times are frequently measured in minutes, an acutely bleeding patient probably benefits most from rapid delivery to a trauma center.

After determining that the patient is in a stable condition, the physician decides to perform a peripheral nerve block to relieve the pain of the broken femur, and to facilitate the placement of a traction splint for reduction of the fracture.

What are the advantages to performing regional anesthetic blocks in the field?

Pain from long bone fractures causes reflex spasm of the muscles that are innervated by the same nerves. In this case, the patient is likely to have quadriceps spasm, which results in displacement of the broken bone ends. In addition to aggravating the pain, which causes a vicious cycle of pain→spasm→pain, the displacement can worsen blood loss from the fractured ends of the bone by disturbing any clots that have formed already. Finally, the hypertension associated with the aggravated pain from an isolated long bone fracture may worsen the bleeding at the site of injury.

Analgesic options in the field include opioids, nitrous oxide/oxygen (Entonox), ketamine and regional anesthetic interventions. Non-steroidal anti-inflammatory drugs (NSAIDs) are not typically employed owing to risk of platelet inhibition. Entonox may be useful for manipulation, splinting and transfer, but is contraindicated in patients with potential pneumothorax or head injury, or where cutting equipment is used for extrication (in view of the combustible oxygen content). Ketamine is a potent analgesic with few cardiorespiratory depressive effects, but can produce dysphoria in larger doses. While opioids are quite popular, the side effects that frequently occur (e.g. sedation and respiratory depression) remain at odds with other important goals in prehospital care, namely maintenance of a patient who is responsive to verbal stimuli, and avoidance of any airway maneuvers or ventilatory support. Opioids are also frequently ineffective – a systematic review of prehospital analgesia by Park *et al.* in 2010 showed that 60–70% of patients still had pain levels of more than three out of ten at 10 minutes after receiving morphine or fentanyl. Taking into account the risks of a small delay in transportation, it is often advantageous and appropriate *in the otherwise stable patient* to perform a low-risk regional analgesic intervention.

What are the safety considerations to performing nerve blocks in the field?

First and foremost, establishing cardiorespiratory stability is critical; as discussed above, there is little to be gained in attempting to provide analgesia when time-sensitive life-saving interventions await the patient in hospital. Regional anesthesia has a place in the field but, to be safe and effective, it must be performed in carefully selected patients.

Second, the neurovascular status must be assessed before and after handling the fractured limb. The capillary refill time should be determined and compared to the uninjured limb. Neurovascular deficit mandates immediate reduction of the deformity, which should be performed after the provision of adequate pain control. Post-reduction neurovascular status should be frequently reassessed.

In this case, it is also important to rule out crush injury of the thigh, as this type of injury places the patient at high risk for compartment syndrome of the thigh.

Which nerve block is appropriate for this patient?

Patients with femoral shaft fracture have severe pain that originates primarily from the injured periosteum. The pattern of innervation of the femur is not entirely clear, but in general is thought to reflect the innervation of the overlying muscles – therefore some combination of femoral, sciatic and obturator nerve blockade is usually indicated. Tondare and Nadkarni (1982) showed that minimal additional analgesics were required for patients with midshaft fractures receiving femoral nerve blockade (i.e. major site of attachment of the quadriceps), whereas patients with proximal or distal femoral fractures required substantial analgesic supplementation to achieve quality pain relief. This likely relates to the relatively higher contribution of sciatic and/or obturator fibers to the periosteum in these latter areas.

The femoral nerve can be blocked at three general anatomical sites: (1) at the nerve itself in the inguinal crease (a traditional femoral nerve block); (2) via a lumbar plexus approach at the posterior flank; and (3) via a fascia iliaca approach several centimeters lateral to the nerve in the proximal thigh. Of these, the fascia iliaca approach has several advantages in the prehospital setting: it requires minimal equipment (a syringe and needle), little sophisticated training, can be performed in the supine position, is associated with very few adverse effects such as nerve or vascular puncture and does not involve motor nerve stimulation that would cause additional pain to the patient.

What equipment is required for a fascia iliaca block in the field?

The block itself is performed using a landmark technique (see below), and therefore does not require the use of a nerve stimulator or ultrasound technology. However, since the patient will be receiving a large (30–40 ml) bolus of local anesthetic, cardiorespiratory monitoring (EKG, NIBP, SpO_2) should be used during the procedure to warn of possible systemic toxicity, however rare.

How is the fascia iliaca block performed?

The fascia iliaca block relies on the medial spread of local anesthetic in the plane between the fascia iliaca and the iliopsoas muscle, thereby achieving blockade of the femoral nerve (Figure 4.1). The femoral nerve is "sandwiched" between these two structures and, with sufficient volume, local anesthetic placed under the fascia iliaca several centimeters lateral to the nerve should reach the target and result in a good block. Some practitioners claim that local anesthetic can spread proximally underneath the inguinal ligament and towards the lumbar plexus, but this has only been shown inconsistently.

With the patient in the supine position, the anterior superior iliac spine and the pubic tubercle are palpated, and a point marked at the juncture of the lateral third and the medial two-thirds of a line connecting the two bony landmarks (Figure 4.2). The needle insertion site is 1–2 cm caudal to that juncture.

Following aseptic skin preparation, a short-bevel or blunt-tipped needle is advanced through the skin and subcutaneous tissue. As the tip passes through the fascia lata and fascia iliaca, two distinct "pops" should be felt. At this point, the needle tip should be located just below the fascia iliaca. After negative aspiration, 30–40 ml of local anesthetic is administered slowly, then the needle withdrawn. The choice of local anesthetic is based on the combined goals of rapid onset and low toxic potential. For these reasons, lidocaine 1.5–2% is often chosen; this allows for quick relief of pain, reduction of the fracture and comfortable transport to the trauma center where additional definitive interventions can be performed prior to the effect

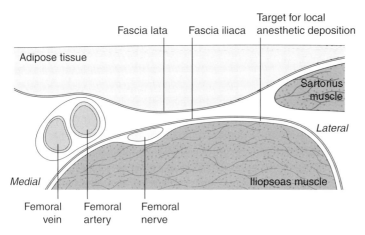

Figure 4.1 Anatomy relevant to the fascia iliaca block. Note the fascia iliaca covering both the iliopsoas muscle and the femoral nerve.

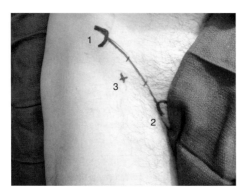

Figure 4.2 Landmarks for the fascia iliaca block. 1, Anterior superior iliac spine; 2, pubic tubercle; 3, mark made 1–2 cm inferior to the junction between the middle two-thirds and the lateral one-third of a line connecting 1 and 2.

wearing off 2–3 hours later. The addition of epinephrine 2.5–5 mcg/ml reduces the peak plasma concentration of local anesthetic and in general prolongs the block when using lidocaine.

In small adults or children, common sense dictates that a weight-based dose be used. Doses ranging from 0.4–0.5 ml/kg have been found to be successful.

What is the success rate using this approach? Are there any adverse effects?

There are only three studies in the published literature on fascia iliaca block in the prehospital setting. None the less, the success rate in significantly reducing pain scores 10 minutes after the block ranged from 94% to 96%. A number of other studies have compared the efficacy of fascia iliaca block compared to standard parenteral opioids in the emergency department setting, with the majority showing an improvement in analgesia and reduction in side effects. Fascia iliaca blocks are by nature quite safe, as there is little to puncture inadvertently. However, one case report (Atchabahian and Brown, 2001) described postoperative neuropathy following a fascia iliaca block performed for postoperative pain; the authors postulated that anatomical variation in the nerve position may have been responsible for this rare outcome.

Is there a role for ultrasound-guided blocks in the field?

Traditionally, ultrasound (US) machines have been designed to be stationary devices used at specific locations in hospital (radiology suite, emergency department, operating room, etc.). However, in recent years, a number of manufacturers have designed relatively low-cost, high-quality portable machines that can be transported and used at the point-of-care, both in-hospital and in the field, for example on EMS vehicles and during military engagements. An example of such a machine is shown in Figure 4.3; this was designed with a view to providing EMS responders with a means to facilitate venous access and perform basic diagnostic assessments, but is also useful for performing peripheral nerve blocks.

The purpose of using US guidance for fascia iliaca block is to ensure that the spread of local anesthetic is beneath the fascial plane. A linear probe is placed over the femoral region in the transverse orientation (Figure 4.4), and the femoral artery and nerve, fascia iliaca and the sartorius muscle identified. The needle is inserted from the lateral side in-plane to puncture the fascia iliaca at a point just deep to the medial aspect of the sartorius muscle (Figure 4.5). The transducer may need to be slid medially to establish that local anesthetic is reaching the femoral nerve, which usually requires 30–40 ml of volume.

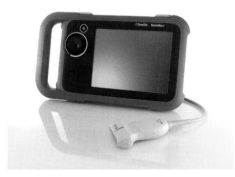

Figure 4.3 Portable ultrasound machine that can be used for field and prehospital use. This unit has durability and simplicity as primary design features. Photo from Sonosite, Inc. with permission.

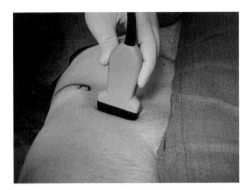

Figure 4.4 Transducer position for an ultrasound-guided fascia iliaca block.

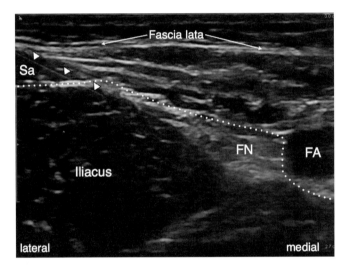

Figure 4.5 Sonoanatomy for the fascia iliaca block. FA, Femoral artery; FN, femoral nerve; Sa, sartorius muscle. The dotted line corresponds to the fascia iliaca. Arrowheads are pointing to the needle, which is positioned just below the fascia iliaca.

Twenty-eight hours later the patient is in the step-down unit following intramedullary nailing of her femur, which was well tolerated with general anesthesia. The nurse calls you and states that over the past several hours the patient has become confused, restless, hypotensive, tachycardic and tachypneic. Her SpO_2 is 92% on 40% O_2.

What is the likely diagnosis? What other features are likely to be present?

In the context of the patient's injury and surgical procedure, the clinical picture is consistent with fat embolism syndrome (FES). FES is a constellation of signs and symptoms that are related to the presence of fat emboli in the bloodstream. Trauma is the principal cause, and high-risk factors include both the movement of unstable long bone fragments and the reaming of medullary cavities. Femoral shaft fractures are particularly prone to developing FES (incidence of 7.6%), compared with 0.3–1.3% for all fractures combined. However, the risk increases with the number of bones fractured.

Table 4.1 Diagnostic criteria for FES

Criteria	Clinical and laboratory features
Gurd and Wilson (One major + four minor + fat microglobulinemia)	Major criteria • Respiratory insufficiency • Cerebral involvement • Petechial rash Minor criteria • Fever • Retinal changes • Tachycardia • Jaundice • Oliguria/anuria • Thrombocytopenia • ↑ESR • Anemia
Schonfeld fat embolism index (≥5 points)	Petechial rash (5 points) Alveolar infiltrates (4 points) Hypoxemia (PO_2 <70 mmHg on 100% O_2) (3 points) Confusion (1 point) Fever (1 point) Tachycardia (1 point) Tachypnea (1 point)
Lindeque (Femur fracture ± tibial fracture + one feature)	PaO_2 <60 mmHg $PaCO_2$ >55 mmHg or pH <7.3 RR >35/min ↑Work of breathing (dyspnea, anxiety, accessory muscle use, etc.)

There is no agreed-upon diagnostic criteria for FES, but several criteria have been proposed (Table 4.1). The classic picture is of a patient with respiratory distress, CNS derangements, pulmonary hypertension and system hypotension, and petechial rash of the upper torso and conjunctiva. Other findings include retinopathy (including retinal fat globules), thrombocytopenia, arrhythmias, oliguria and myocardial ischemia.

What is the pathophysiology of fat embolism syndrome?

There are two principal theories explaining the pathologic and clinical manifestations of FES. Both begin with fat from bone marrow entering the circulation through venous sinusoids (e.g. after injury or reaming), thereby producing microscopic emboli. The two theories then differ as follows.

- **Mechanical hypothesis:** this theory states that the accumulated fat emboli act as a mechanical obstruction to bloodflow, both in the pulmonary system (causing pulmonary hypertension) and in the systemic circulation, which accounts for the CNS, skin and other organ changes. The principal weakness of this theory is that it fails to explain the 24–72-hour interval between injury and onset of the syndrome that is frequently seen.

- **Biochemical hypothesis:** this theory states that fat in the blood is degraded to toxic intermediaries, including free fatty acids and C-reactive protein, which then go on to cause injury to multiple organ systems. This theory explains the delay in symptoms, as it takes some time for fat to be degraded in the plasma.

It is likely that both mechanisms play a role in the variable picture seen in FES.

How is fat embolism syndrome treated?

Treatment of FES is supportive, including oxygen therapy, ventilatory and hemodynamic support and intravenous fluids. Corticosteroids have been shown in some trials to benefit patients, but firm evidence supporting this is lacking. Despite the need for advanced resuscitation, the overall mortality is low and most patients recover fully.

Early immobilization of fractures has been shown to reduce the incidence of FES. The longer the period of time for which the broken ends of the long bone are displaced and prone to mechanical disruption, the higher the risk of fat emboli. This lends support to the decision in this case to reduce the displaced fracture in the field with the aid of a fascia iliaca block.

References and further reading

Akhtar, S. (2009). Fat embolism. *Anesthesiology Clinics*, **27**, 533–50.

Atchabahian, A., Brown, A. R. (2001). Postoperative neuropathy following fascia iliaca compartment blockade. *Anesthesiology*, **94**, 534–6.

Aydin, S., Overwater, E., Saltzherr, T. P. *et al.* (2010). The association of mobile medical team involvement on on-scene times and mortality in trauma patients. *The Journal of Trauma*, **69**, 589–94.

Border, J. R., Lewis, F. R., Aprahamian, C. *et al.* (1983). Panel: prehospital trauma care–stabilize or scoop and run. *The Journal of Trauma*, **23**, 708–11.

Gozlan, C., Minville, V., Asehnoune, K. *et al.* (2005). [Fascia iliaca block for femoral bone fractures in prehospital medicine]. *Annales Françaises D'anesthèsie Et De Rèanimation*, **24**, 617–20.

Lopez, S., Gros, T., Bernard, N., Plasse, C., Capdevila, X. (2003). Fascia iliaca compartment block for femoral bone fractures in prehospital care. *Regional Anesthesia and Pain Medicine*, **28**, 203–7.

Minville, V., Gozlan, C., Asehnoune, K. *et al.* (2006). Fascia-iliaca compartment block for femoral bone fracture in prehospital medicine in a 6-yr-old child. *European Journal of Anaesthesiology*, **23**, 715–16.

Nirula, R., Maier, R., Moore, E., Sperry, J., Gentilello, L. (2010). Scoop and run to the trauma center or stay and play at the local hospital: hospital transfer's effect on mortality. *The Journal of Trauma*, **69**, 595–9.

Park, C. L., Roberts, D. E., Aldington, D. J., Moore, R. A. (2010). Prehospital analgesia: systematic review of evidence. *Journal of the Royal Army Medical Corps*, **156**, 295–300.

Riska, E. B., Myllynen, P. (1982). Fat embolism in patients with multiple injuries. *The Journal of Trauma*, **22**, 891–4.

Timmermann, A., Russo, S. G., Hollmann, M. W. (2008). Paramedic versus emergency physician emergency medical service: role of the anaesthesiologist and the European versus the Anglo-American concept. *Current Opinion in Anaesthesiology*, **21**, 222–7.

Tondare, A. S., Nadkarni, A. V. (1982). Femoral nerve block for fractured shaft of femur. *Canadian Anaesthetists' Society Journal*, **29**, 270–1.

Regional anesthesia and digital replantation

Key aspects of case

1. Advantages of regional anesthesia for digital replantation surgery.
2. Use of long-term brachial plexus catheters for repeat procedures and pain management in the ICU.
3. Perineural catheter site infection.

Case presentation

A 17-year-old male is brought to hospital following an accident on his family farm where his hand was caught in the fan blades of a tractor he was trying to fix. He is conscious and able to converse, but is extremely anxious. His right hand is bandaged with blood-soaked gauze, and the ambulance crew states that his thumb almost completely severed through the thenar eminence and is just "hanging by a thread of tissue" (Figure 5.1). They estimate approximately 500 ml of blood loss in the field, and no other associated injuries. He is healthy otherwise, has no allergies and takes no medications. His last meal was 2 hours ago. Vitals are BP 151/86 mmHg, HR 102 bpm, RR 22/min, temperature 36.5°C and SpO$_2$ 99% on facemask oxygen. He is scheduled to be transferred urgently to the operating room for debridement and replantation of the digit.

Case discussion

What are the key considerations for limb or digital replantation?

The principal goals of upper limb, hand or finger replantation are to restore circulation and to regain enough function and sensation in the amputated part so as to facilitate return to previous employment and/or activities of daily living. Amputation injuries can be broadly classified into three types based on mechanism: clean-cut (guillotine), crush and avulsion injuries. Of these, the first type has the best prognosis for functional recovery, whereas the latter two often have poor results. Since the thumb is responsible for 40% of hand function, this digit is always given first priority for replantation; in cases where the thumb cannot be replanted, the least damaged finger should be transposed to the thumb position. Single digit amputations of the second through fifth finger are generally not replanted as functional impairment is minimal.

Several other factors affect the outcome of replanted digits, hands and limbs. Avoidance of prolonged ischemia is particularly important for muscle tissue, and therefore is a more

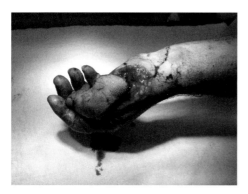

Figure 5.1 Near amputation of the left thumb.

pertinent concern for whole limbs compared to digits, which lack muscle. Permitted warm ischemia time for a limb is approximately 6 h, compared to 12 h for digits. Cooling the amputated digit increases allowable ischemic time to up to 30 h. Patient factors that adversely affect the circulation, such as cigarette smoking, connective tissue disease, diabetes mellitus and atherosclerosis, all reduce the likelihood of successful replant.

The order in which structures are repaired during digital replantation is: bone, tendons, arteries, veins and nerves.

What are the initial steps in management of digital amputation?

Initial evaluation and resuscitation should conform to advanced trauma life support (ATLS) guidelines, and life-threatening injuries should be identified and treated. For complete amputations, the amputated part should be wrapped in moist gauze and placed in a plastic bag, which is then immersed in a cooler with an ice pack, or an ice-water bath. In cases of incomplete amputation such as this one, tissue bridges should be preserved if possible. Following wrapping of the injured region with moist gauze, ice packs are placed around the distal portion. Radiographs are taken to determine the extent of skeletal injury.

Control of bleeding is an early priority and should be accomplished by direct pressure to the gauze-wrapped limb. An elastic bandage can be gently wrapped around the proximal stump to prevent further blood loss. Ultimately, expedient transfer to an operating room for examination of the area, hemostasis, debridement and microsurgical replantation is the definitive therapy.

What are the anesthetic considerations and goals of managing patients undergoing replantation?

1. **Time**: replantations are generally time-consuming procedures, with multiple digital replants often taking up to 12–18 h or longer. In cases where a patient has poor medical fitness, a discussion with the surgeon is warranted regarding the risks/benefits of proceeding with the operation.

2. **Vasospasm/thrombosis**: these potentially catastrophic events can lead to loss of the replanted digit. Interventions to reduce the risk of these include the maintenance of strict normothermia once the arterial anastomosis begins, avoidance of vasoconstrictor agents

such as phenylephrine or metaraminol, maintenance of the hematocrit at approximately 30% to improve viscosity and microcirculation, and sympatholysis by the use of sympathetic or brachial plexus blocks. In addition, most microsurgical teams use some combination of aspirin, heparin and dextran to counteract the hypercoagulable response to trauma.

3. **Pain control**: quality analgesia with regional anesthesia plus a multimodal adjuvant regimen will decrease the stress response and reduce the risk of thrombosis and vasospasm.

What are the anesthetic options for this case?

Because of the frequent prolonged nature of these procedures and the frequent need for vein and/or skin graft harvesting from other sites, regional anesthesia alone is often impractical. For the reasons stated above, many anesthesiologists elect to provide general anesthesia with concurrent brachial plexus or forearm catheters for both pain control and to produce a chemical sympathectomy.

What are the options for postoperative analgesia?

All patients should receive multimodal analgesia, including acetaminophen plus NSAIDs or cyclo-oxygenase (COX)-2 inhibitors, unless contraindicated. Opioids may be used for break-though pain. However, the highest quality analgesia is provided by continuous peripheral nerve block at the brachial plexus. Besides rendering the surgical site insensate, the sympathectomy provided serves to combat any neurogenic vasospasm that may otherwise occur. Likewise, blocking afferent nociceptive signals with a continuous nerve catheter reduces the release of counter-regulatory hormones, catecholamines and acute phase reactants that all contribute to a detrimental stress response. While a single-shot nerve block provides excellent pain relief in the short term, the time period during which these patients are at risk for vasospasm and thrombosis (and hence require sympathectomy) lasts for several days postoperatively.

Catheters placed at any site along the brachial plexus can be expected to provide adequate hand analgesia; theoretically the interscalene approach has been considered less attractive because of concerns over sparing of the inferior trunk, but this can be overcome with the use of ultrasonography and the precise placement of the catheter near the middle and lower trunks. Disadvantages of placing a catheter at the axilla relate to problems maintaining sterility and its dislodgement potential owing to skin mobility. The infraclavicular and supraclavicular approaches are both consistently reliable for hand analgesia. Many practitioners find that infraclavicular catheters are less likely to become dislodged compared to supraclavicular catheters owing to the greater depth and the fact that the catheter passes through 0.5–2 cm of pectoralis muscle, which may aid in "gripping" the catheter and preventing accidental withdrawal.

What are the considerations regarding anticoagulation and brachial plexus catheters?

Most post-replant patients will receive multiple anticoagulants, including a heparinoid, aspirin and/or dextran for several days. Little evidence exists to guide decision-making for placement of peripheral nerve catheters in the anticoagulated patient, and the issue remains controversial. Most experts agree that placement of catheters at a site that is both superficial and easily compressible (e.g. axillary brachial plexus) represents a low risk profile. However, inadvertent vascular puncture at a deeper and less accessible site (e.g. during infraclavicular block) may result in clinically significant bleeding, especially when 18- or 19-gauge catheter insertion needles are used. Ultrasonography has changed the threshold for performing infraclavicular blocks in anticoagulated patients, and it is no longer considered a contraindication, especially when the benefits of a long-term catheter are numerous, as is the case with this patient. Careful pre-procedure scanning and identification of the relevant vasculature and plexus structures is essential prior to insertion of the needle.

A right infraclavicular brachial plexus catheter is placed using ultrasound guidance. Twenty millilitres of 0.25% ropivacaine is injected via the catheter and can be visualized spreading well immediately deep to the axillary artery.

What are the technical considerations in placing an ultrasound-guided infraclavicular catheter?

- Abducting the arm 90° decreases the distance from the skin to the plexus and improves visualization of the neurovascular structures

- In thin patients, a linear transducer is often adequate for visualization. However, a curved array transducer will provide better images for patients with substantial chest wall muscle or fat, and may improve needle visualization. The transducer position (Figure 5.2) is immediately medial to the coracoid process and caudad to the clavicle in the parasagittal orientation

- Color Doppler should be used to identify the axillary artery, axillary vein and cephalic vein (Figure 5.3), and to plan the needle trajectory

- A 10-cm catheter insertion needle should be introduced from the cephalad aspect and advanced towards the posterior cord, which lies deep to the axillary artery. Frequent administration of 0.5–1 ml of injectate (hydrodissection) aids in locating the needle tip if the needle is not readily visible

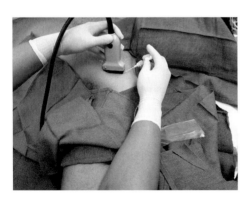

Figure 5.2 Transducer and needle position for ultrasound-guided continuous infraclavicular brachial plexus block.

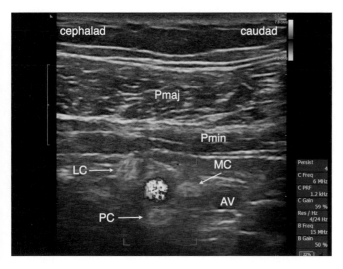

Figure 5.3 Sonoanatomy for the infraclavicular block. The neurovascular structures are located deep to both pectoralis major (Pmaj) and minor (Pmin) muscles. The lateral cord (LC), posterior cord (PC) and medial cord (MC) can be seen clustered around the axillary artery. The color Doppler function is being used to help identify the artery. The axillary vein (AV) is seen caudal to the medial cord.

- Nerve stimulation may be difficult to interpret in cases of complete digital amputation, when forced to rely on a forearm or wrist extensor response. Nerve stimulation may in fact be potentially harmful in cases of incomplete amputation
- The catheter should only be advanced 1–2 cm beyond the tip of the needle to avoid catheter knotting and/or an increased final nerve-to-catheter distance
- Confirmation of catheter tip location is best achieved with the Doppler function or the use of a small amount of agitated air/fluid injectate. Witnessed "blush" at the 6 o'clock position relative to the axillary artery predicts a successful block.

What are the local anesthetic choices and infusion regimen options?

The goals for this infusion regimen are to:

- Provide analgesia and sympathectomy without motor blockade
- Titrate the analgesic effect to pain of varying intensity such as dressing changes or repeat surgical procedures
- Minimize local anesthetic consumption to reduce risk of systemic toxicity.

For brachial plexus blocks, this is best accomplished with a background infusion (5–8 ml/h) of ropivacaine 2%, plus a patient-controlled bolus (4–8 ml) every 20–60 minutes. Bupivacaine is not commonly used owing to concerns regarding systemic toxicity, as well as the increased incidence of motor block compared to ropivacaine. Lidocaine is a relatively safe local anesthetic but, in concentrations required to provide analgesia, this drug also contributes to an increase in motor blockade.

Adjuvants such as clonidine and epinephrine have little role in improving analgesia in continuous catheter techniques. In this particular case, epinephrine should be used with care owing to its vasoconstrictive properties in the digital vessels. Clonidine has only been shown to increase the incidence of motor block in continuous peripheral nerve blocks.

How long can brachial plexus catheters be left in place? What are the risks and benefits?

Choosing an appropriate duration for perineural infusion requires weighing the benefit of continued analgesia and sympathectomy against the risk of complications. Most perineural catheters remain *in situ* for 2–5 days, but in cases where patients require extended medical transport or prolonged sympathetic blockade, durations in excess of 4–12 weeks have been reported. This patient may require serial surgical procedures (e.g. dressing changes, debridement) over 1–2 weeks, and the catheter may be kept *in situ* until recovery is assured and the risk of vascular complications at the graft site has subsided.

Technical problems such as catheter knotting, breakage and shearing can occur. However, the most worrisome complications include local anesthetic systemic toxicity, neurologic injury and infection. The risks of systemic toxicity and neurologic injury are difficult to quantify, but appear to be very rare. For example, the risk of nerve injury lasting longer than 9 months associated with continuous nerve blocks is estimated at 0.07%. Risk of infection is related to duration of catheter placement, and, while rates of catheter colonization may exceed 50%, clinically relevant infection has an overall reported incidence of <1%.

What are the risk factors for developing a perineural catheter-related infection?

1. **Trauma**: suggested causes include a greater range of bacterial skin flora and/or difficulties in maintaining asepsis during catheter placement in trauma patients.

2. **Intensive care admission**: this may be related to impaired cellular immunity and upregulated inflammatory response in the critical care setting.

3. **Duration of perineural catheter infusion > 48 hours**.

4. **Absence of antibiotic prophylaxis**: a single dose at the time of insertion may not be sufficient to prevent infection and ongoing prophylaxis is generally warranted.

5. **Site of insertion**: femoral and axillary catheters are associated with a higher rate of colonization than interscalene or popliteal sciatic catheters. This may be because of the high concentration of sebaceous glands in these areas, which reduces the effectiveness of disinfectant solutions to adhere to the skin.

6. **Male sex**: this is likely related to the population most at risk for trauma.

Further reading

Beris, A. E., Lykissas, M. G., Korompilias, A. V. *et al.* (2010). Digit and hand replantation. *Archives of Orthopaedic and Trauma Surgery*, **130**, 1141–7.

Bigeleisen, P. E. (2007). Ultrasound-guided infraclavicular block in an anticoagulated and anesthetized patient. *Anesthesia and Analgesia*, **104**, 1285–7.

Capdevila, X., Bringuier, S., Borgeat, A. (2009). Infectious risk of continuous peripheral nerve blocks. *Anesthesiology*, **110**, 182–8.

Caplan, R. A., Long, M. C. (1984). Prolonged anesthesia – management and sequelae of a two-day general anesthetic. *Anesthesia and Analgesia*, **63**, 353–8.

Hebl, J. R. (2006). The importance and implications of aseptic techniques during regional anesthesia. *Regional Anesthesia and Pain Medicine*, **31**, 311–23.

Ilfeld, B. M. (2011). Review article: continuous peripheral nerve blocks: a review of the published evidence. *Anesthesia and Analgesia*, **113**, 904–25.

Shanahan, P. T. (1984). Replantation anesthesia. *Anesthesia and Analgesia*, **63**, 785–6.

Taras, J. S., Behrman, M. J. (1998). Continuous peripheral nerve block in replantation and revascularization. *Journal of Reconstructive Microsurgery*, **14**, 17–21.

Chapter 6

Regional anesthesia and compartment syndrome

Key aspects of case

1. Analgesic management of the patient at risk for compartment syndrome, including considerations for single injection versus continuous perineural catheter techniques.
2. Monitoring of the patient at risk for compartment syndrome.

Case presentation

A 29-year-old male is brought to hospital after being struck by a taxi while crossing a busy intersection on his bicycle. The paramedics report that he was conscious at the scene, but somewhat dazed, and was wearing a helmet at the time of the impact. His vital signs are BP 154/86, HR 99, RR 20 and SpO$_2$ 99% on facemask oxygen. He is alert and responding to commands appropriately. A survey of his injuries reveals multiple skin abrasions, several superficial lacerations on his upper extremities, and a closed left proximal tibial fracture. He states that he is "sore all over," but he has no other obvious injuries. The orthopedic surgeon evaluates the patient and books him for an intramedullary nailing of the tibia to be performed the following morning.

Case discussion

What are the key issues in the management of tibial fractures?

The tibia is the most commonly fractured long bone in the body, and this injury is usually associated with high-speed trauma such as that incurred in motor vehicle accidents or high-velocity sporting activities (e.g. skiing). As such, the patient should be carefully evaluated for other concomitant injuries. Other key considerations are the presence of open wounds at the fracture site and neurovascular insufficiency. While all open fractures should be treated operatively, some closed fractures are amenable to closed reduction and immobilization, depending on the degree of instability. One of the most serious concerns is the potential for acute compartment syndrome (ACS) following injuries (either fractures or soft tissue) to the leg, and a high index of suspicion is required for this complication. The operative treatment of choice is usually the placement of an intramedullary nail, as it is associated with fewer infectious complications and less soft-tissue trauma than the plating of the fracture. In cases where IM nailing might be challenging, or in severely comminuted fractures, external fixation can be used.

What is the pathophysiology of ACS? Why is the leg prone to the development of ACS?

ACS occurs when the pressure within a closed compartment rises above capillary perfusion pressure, compromising the circulation and tissue function within that space. When the capillaries collapse, flow through the tissue beds and into the venous system ceases, leading to tissue hypoxia and the release of mediators increasing vascular permeability. The resultant leakage of fluid through capillary and muscle membranes increases edema and worsens the intracompartmental pressure, leading to a vicious cycle of increased pressure → ischemia → leakage → increased pressure. Normal tissue pressure is usually 0–10 mmHg, and capillary filling pressure is equivalent to diastolic arterial pressure. When the gradient between tissue pressure and diastolic blood pressure falls to within 30 mmHg, risk for capillary collapse and development of ACS rises significantly.

The leg is divided into four distinct anatomic compartments containing specific muscles, nerves and vessels (Figure 6.1). Each compartment is bounded by inelastic osteo-fascial planes that do not permit expansion in the event of an increase in intra-compartmental volume (e.g. trauma, bleeding or swelling). The anterior compartment

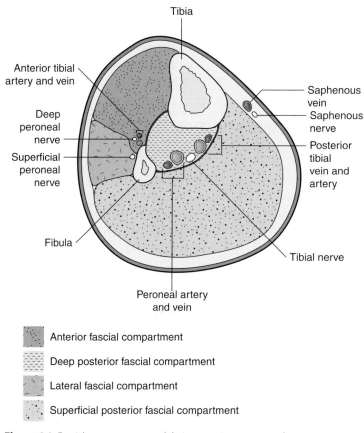

Anterior fascial compartment

Deep posterior fascial compartment

Lateral fascial compartment

Superficial posterior fascial compartment

Figure 6.1 Fascial compartments and their respective neurovascular structures.

contains the dorsiflexors of the foot, the deep peroneal nerve and the anterior tibial artery and vein; the lateral compartment contains the foot evertors (peroneus longus and brevis), as well as the superficial peroneal nerve; the deep posterior compartment houses the plantar flexors, as well as both the posterior tibial and peroneal vessels; finally, the superficial posterior compartment contains the large plantar flexors (gastrocnemius and soleus), but no vessels or nerves. Of these, the anterior compartment is the one most frequently affected by ACS, although in the case of high-velocity injuries such as this one, multiple compartments are often involved.

What is the epidemiology of acute compartment syndrome?

The average annual incidence of ACS for western nations is approximately 3 per 100 000. Over one-third of all cases of ACS are associated with tibial fracture, particularly the proximal and middle thirds of the diaphysis (because of the bulkier muscle mass compared with the distal leg). Other common fracture sites leading to ACS include diaphyseal fractures of the forearm and distal radius fractures. Older reports suggested that supracondylar fractures in children were also a high-risk injury, but this is less commonly seen in current practice, and the discrepancy may be caused by outdated hyperflexion casting practices. The second most common cause after fracture is blunt soft-tissue injury. Multiple other causes exist, such as crush or reperfusion injury, exercise, arterial puncture, circumferential dressings, burns and snake bites. Younger age (<35 years) is a risk factor, increasing the incidence of ACS following tibial fracture by 30-fold, and males outnumber females by approximately 10:1. There appears to be no difference in ACS rates following open versus closed fractures.

Compartment syndrome also occurs in the upper arm, thigh, foot, hand, buttock and abdomen.

How is the diagnosis of ACS made?

The diagnosis of ACS has traditionally been a clinical one, based primarily on the presence of pain out of proportion and paresthesia. Despite clinicians' reliance on these symptoms, they have been shown to be quite variable and largely unreliable. Pain may be minimal or absent if nerve injury is present. Tense, swollen fascial compartments and pain on passive stretching are often present, but not always. Paralysis is a late sign and is often irreversible. Pulselessness and pallor are frequently described, but are in fact rare, as the pressures that cause ACS are usually well below systemic arterial pressure. The few studies that have investigated the utility of clinical signs and symptoms have shown a sensitivity and positive predictive value of only 11–15%, while the specificity and negative predictive value were 97–98%. In other words, the classic clinical findings are more likely to be present in a patient *without* ACS than in a patient with the syndrome; on the other hand, an absence of clinical signs and symptoms is a reassuring sign. These signs are clearly even less useful in the sedated or neurologically impaired patient.

The unreliability of clinical signs has prompted some major trauma intensive care units to abandon physical examination as part of the screening process for ACS, and instead rely solely on objective measurements of compartmental pressures (Figure 6.2) or tissue ischemia (Table 6.1).

Table 6.1 Non-clinical monitors for compartment syndrome

Monitor	Method	Notes
Compartment pressure monitoring	Needle manometers are placed in individual compartments and pressure recorded Normal pressure 10–12 mmHg Absolute tissue pressures have been used (i.e. 30–45 mmHg), but may underestimate risk in hypotension ΔP (diastolic pressure–tissue pressure) of 30 mmHg probably more reliable	Cheap and easy Can be used continuously, but are prone to clotting/blockage Should be performed as close to the site of fracture as possible; a 10 mmHg reduction in tissue pressure is expected for every 5 cm distal that the pressure is measured
Near infrared spectroscopy (NIRS)	Measures tissue oxygenation (StO₂) Values strongly reflect compartmental pressure, perfusion pressure and loss of muscle function	Non-invasive, can be used continuously Expensive Only useful for shallow (i.e. surface) compartments; not able to measure deep posterior compartment of calf
Creatine phosphokinase	Estimates degree of muscle damage	Cheap, nearly always available Late indicator, damage has already started to occur May be confusing in polytrauma where there are other sources of damaged muscle

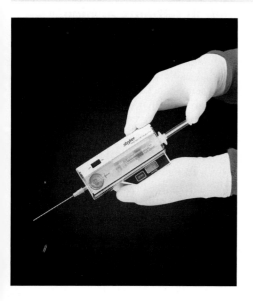

Figure 6.2 A portable intracompartmental pressure monitor (Stryker Instruments, Kalamazoo, MI). This hand-held disposable device allows for rapid and accurate bedside quantification of compartmental pressures. With permission from Stryker Instruments.

What is the treatment for ACS?

Compartment syndrome is a surgical emergency and requires immediate fasciotomy to reduce the tissue pressure in the affected compartments. In general, two longitudinal incisions are made, one laterally and one medially, to decompress all four fascial compartments.

The patient is to be admitted for overnight observation prior to his procedure in the morning. In the meantime, he is complaining of 9/10 pain at the site of fracture despite 24 mg of intravenous morphine and is requesting additional pain relief.

How might a regional block interfere with the diagnosis of ACS?

Despite the evidence demonstrating that clinical signs are unreliable, many clinicians still rely on the presence or absence of pain as a diagnostic tool for ACS. In the past, patients were frequently denied quality analgesia for fear of missing the "cardinal" signs and symptoms of ACS. This fear has led many surgeons and anesthesiologists to advocate against the use of neuraxial and peripheral nerve blocks in this population. While there are relatively few reports of the use of regional blockade in the setting of ACS, epidural analgesia has been implicated in the delayed diagnosis of ACS in three patients, all of whom had dense bilateral motor blocks for more than 18 hours after their operations. A common finding in these three cases was a lack of breakthrough pain because of their profound sensory and motor blockade. Other prospective audits of epidural analgesia suggest that neuraxial analgesia helped to facilitate the diagnosis owing to increasing severity of breakthrough pain.

The evidence for peripheral nerve blocks (PNBs) is more encouraging – there is no evidence that PNBs delay diagnosis of upper limb or thigh compartment syndrome. There are a small number of reports that attribute delays in diagnosis to lower limb nerve blocks, but the mechanism is somewhat incongruous (e.g. a femoral nerve block delaying diagnosis of calf compartment syndrome).

Should regional anesthesia be avoided in patients at high risk for ACS?

Patients who are traumatically injured deserve quality pain control. While opioids (and other multimodal non-opioid analgesics) have their place in acute pain management, the gold standard for isolated acute limb pain is peripheral nerve blockade. It provides superior analgesia to opioids, particularly when given by a continuous catheter technique, and carries fewer side effects than either opioids or epidural analgesia.

There is no literature to support the view that opioids are inherently safer than regional anesthesia in this setting. In fact, there are at least six reports of delayed diagnosis of ACS attributable to opioid analgesia. However, this is not the principal issue, as no patient should be denied access to quality pain control. Instead, the question should be: "If a patient is at high risk for ACS, should they not be monitored *objectively*, rather than clinically, for this complication?" Instead of excluding an extremely effective analgesic modality such as regional analgesia, a decision should be made by the care team early to initiate compartmental pressure monitoring or near infrared spectroscopy. At the same time, a rational strategy can be employed for the use of regional analgesia that mitigates the risk of delayed diagnosis.

How can the risk of delayed diagnosis of ACS be minimized while using regional anesthesia/analgesia?

Two general strategies can be used to minimize the risk of delayed diagnosis. First, and most importantly, dilute solutions of local anesthesia must be used for analgesia. There is no requirement for a profound motor block in the preoperative or postoperative setting. Moreover, a dilute solution has been shown in multiple reports to actually facilitate the *early* diagnosis of ACS if and when the patient reports progressive breakthrough pain. The ischemic pain of ACS is difficult to mask with dilute analgesic solutions of local anesthetic, and requires surgical anesthetic concentrations to control. Examples of appropriately dilute solutions are ropivacaine 0.1–0.2%, or bupivacaine/levobupivacaine 0.1–0.125%. It is appropriate to use epidural opioids as well in dilute concentrations (e.g. fentanyl 2–4 mcg/ml), and these do not contribute to a motor block.

The second strategy is the use of continuous peripheral nerve catheter techniques. The placement of a sciatic catheter is a common intervention for tibial shaft fractures at our institution. Their advantage lies in the clinician's ability to alter the concentration of the local anesthetic to match the intervention (surgical procedure versus postoperative pain) or to stop the infusion entirely if required. Catheters can be placed at any time during the hospital course and left "dry" (or with a small infusion of saline to prevent clotting), and then bolused when appropriate. When possible, dilute solutions of local anesthetics (e.g. ropivacaine 0.2%) should be used.

A popliteal sciatic catheter is placed and the patient started on an infusion of ropivacaine 0.2% at 5 ml/h, with a bolus feature of 5 ml every 30 minutes. The patient expresses his gratitude for the improved pain control, and is sent to the floor. All is quiet until 4 a.m., when you receive a call from the nursing staff stating that the patient is complaining of increased pain in the leg.

How do you assess the patient and what are your initial interventions?

Since the patient is at high risk for ACS, this requires immediate attention. The patient should be queried about the timing, location and nature of the pain, and the infusion pump interrogated to assess local anesthetic usage. Physical examination of the leg, including palpation of calf compartments and measurement of calf circumference, should be performed; however, in this situation, establishment of compartmental pressures is indicated and this should be performed by a physician experienced in this type of monitoring.

Compartment and perfusion pressures are found to be normal and, several hours later, the patient is brought to the operating room for intramedullary nailing of the fracture. He is still receiving the ropivacaine 0.2% infusion.

What are the anesthetic options?

In this situation, there are essentially three options: general anesthesia, neuraxial anesthesia and PNB using the *in-situ* catheter. There may be existing concerns that make the induction of general anesthesia less appealing (e.g. potential cervical spine injury, full stomach, etc.). On the other hand, many trauma patients simply cannot lie still for 2 hours while a procedure is performed under regional block. Neuraxial anesthesia may be effective, but may be challenging to perform in a patient who is unable to position himself ideally owing to generalized pain. If a neuraxial technique is chosen, consideration to the duration of lower extremity block should be made, although it is unlikely that a compartment syndrome would develop in the first 2–3 hours immediately following the operation.

If the sciatic catheter is functioning well, this may be a good option. The local anesthetic of choice for surgical anesthesia in this case should be short- or intermediate-acting (i.e. high concentrations of either ropivacaine or bupivacaine should be avoided). Lidocaine 2% or mepivacaine 1.5% are appropriate choices, and will provide 3–4 hours of surgical anesthesia. After the procedure, the infusion of dilute ropivacaine or bupivacaine can be reinitiated.

Further reading

Al-Hadithy, N., Al-Nammari, S. (2010). Towards evidence based emergency medicine: best BETs from the Manchester Royal Infirmary. BET 4. Positioning of compartment pressure monitors in lower limb fractures. *Emergency Medicine Journal: EMJ*, **27**, 954–5.

Davis, E. T., Harris, A., Keene, D., Porter, K., Manji, M. (2006). The use of regional anaesthesia in patients at risk of acute compartment syndrome. *Injury*, **37**, 128–33.

Garr, J. L., Gentilello, L. M., Cole, P. A., Mock, C. N., Matsen, F. A., 3rd. (1999). Monitoring for compartmental syndrome using near-infrared spectroscopy: a noninvasive, continuous, transcutaneous monitoring technique. *The Journal of Trauma*, **46**, 613–16.

Harrington, P., Bunola, J., Jennings, A. J., Bush, D. J., Smith, R. M. (2000). Acute compartment syndrome masked by intravenous morphine from a patient-controlled analgesia pump. *Injury*, **31**, 387–9.

Hocking, G. (2007). Re: The use of regional anaesthesia in patients at risk of acute compartment syndrome. *Injury*, **38**, 872–3.

Kakar, S., Firoozabadi, R., McKean, J., Tornetta, P., 3rd. (2007). Diastolic blood pressure in patients with tibia fractures under anaesthesia: implications for the diagnosis of compartment syndrome. *Journal of Orthopaedic Trauma*, **21**, 99–103.

Karagiannis, G., Hardern, R. (2005). Best evidence topic report. No evidence found that a femoral nerve block in cases of femoral shaft fractures can delay the diagnosis of compartment syndrome of the thigh. *Emergency Medicine Journal: EMJ*, **22**, 814.

Kosir, R., Moore, F. A., Selby, J. H. *et al.* (2007). Acute lower extremity compartment syndrome (ALECS) screening protocol in critically ill trauma patients. *The Journal of Trauma*, **63**, 268–75.

Mar, G. J., Barrington, M. J., McGuirk, B. R. (2009). Acute compartment syndrome of the lower limb and the effect of postoperative analgesia on diagnosis. *British Journal of Anaesthesia*, **102**, 3–11.

Masquelet, A.-C. (2010). Acute compartment syndrome of the leg: pressure measurement and fasciotomy. *Orthopaedics & Traumatology, Surgery & Research: OTSR*, **96**, 913–17.

McQueen, M. M., Gaston, P., Court-Brown, C. M. (2000). Acute compartment syndrome. Who is at risk? *The Journal of Bone and Joint Surgery. British Volume*, **82**, 200–3.

Ulmer, T. (2002). The clinical diagnosis of compartment syndrome of the lower leg: are clinical findings predictive of the disorder? *Journal of Orthopaedic Trauma*, **16**, 572–7.

Regional anesthesia for blunt chest trauma

Key aspects of case

1. Prevention of pulmonary complications with regional analgesic techniques (intercostal, paravertebral, epidural, intrapleural) following blunt thoracic trauma.
2. Considerations regarding local anesthetic systemic toxicity.

Case presentation

A 47-year-old female police officer is brought to hospital by a colleague after being thrown from her horse while on assignment patrolling a student demonstration. She is awake and alert, with a GCS of 15, but complaining of pain over her left anterolateral chest, where she struck a guardrail. Examination reveals a patent airway, bilateral breath sounds and no evidence of external bleeding or penetrating chest injury. Her vital signs are HR 98, BP 141/92, RR 28 and SpO₂ 95% on facemask oxygen. She is neurologically intact and has full range of motion of her cervical spine with no tenderness to palpation. Palpation of her left anterolateral chest is very painful, and a CT scan of her chest reveals a moderate left-sided pulmonary contusion (represent- ing approximately 15% of the airspace) and midshaft fractures of ribs 5 through 8.

Case discussion

What is the pathophysiology of pulmonary contusion?

Pulmonary contusion is a common finding after blunt chest trauma, particularly after falls and the rapid deceleration associated with motor vehicle crashes. The two most significant predictors of pulmonary contusion are an instantaneous change in velocity >45 mph, and a frontal or near-side lateral impact with a fixed object. Alveoli underlying the chest wall are disrupted primarily from the shock wave, or are sheared from heavier hilar tissues because of differing rates of deceleration. The result is interstitial and alveolar bleeding, edema, inflammation and decreased surfactant production, leading to various degrees of hypoxemia, hypercarbia, decreased lung compliance, increased work of breathing, hemoptysis and respiratory failure. The clinical picture peaks at about 72 hours, and in general most patients recover fully with no residual respiratory disease.

How does imaging help in the diagnosis of pulmonary contusion?

Chest X-ray findings of consolidation typically appear 4–6 h after the injury and disappear after several days. However, many chest X-rays taken as part of the trauma workup will miss an evolving process, and tend to underestimate the eventual incidence. CT scanning of the chest is very sensitive; approximately one-third of patients with CT findings of pulmonary contusion after blunt thoracic trauma will not have findings on plain films. CT scanning is also useful in risk stratification as to the need for mechanical ventilation, and for increasing the sensitivity of diagnosing rib fractures compared to plain films.

What is the effect on outcome of multiple rib fractures?

Mortality is known to be linearly associated with the number of ribs fractured, rising from about 10% for three ribs to >30% for six or more ribs. Morbidity increases dramatically if there is concomitant pulmonary contusion. For example, the incidence of respiratory failure is about 20% with rib fracture alone, but 50% if rib fracture is accompanied by pulmonary contusion.

Fractured ribs are markers of injury severity, particularly in younger patients with more pliable rib cages, as more energy is required to cause the injury. Sharp fragments of bone can lacerate underlying organs such as pleura, lung, spleen and liver. Rib fractures are very painful, limiting the patient's ability to breathe deeply, cough and receive physiotherapy, leading to atelectasis, hypoxemia, pneumonia and respiratory distress. Analgesia for rib fractures is clearly a priority in these patients.

What are the advantages and disadvantages of different analgesic modalities for thoracic trauma?

The analgesic plan for thoracic trauma patients should be individualized, as there is no one best modality for all patients. The goals should be to minimize respiratory depression, optimize respiratory excursion while not impairing the uninjured side, and to minimize any possible side effects of the intervention such as local anesthetic systemic toxicity (LAST) or iatrogenic pneumothorax. In addition, the plan should be the simplest one possible that achieves these goals. Examples of possible modalities are outlined in Table 7.1.

Thoracic epidural analgesia (TEA) is the best option for bilateral rib fractures, provided no contraindications exist (e.g. spinal injury). Intercostal blocks are effective, but require multiple injections, are of intermediate duration and carry a risk of pneumothorax (1.5% per block performed). This last concern is obviated if a chest tube is in place. Paravertebral blockade (PVB) is the preferred technique at our institution as it is relatively free from side effects, is easy to perform, can be used with a catheter technique and provides equivalent analgesia to TEA. Systemic opioids have a role in trauma, especially in the patient with multiple injuries who requires urgent surgery followed by a stay in the ICU; however, it is worthwhile supplementing this with a regional technique as soon as their status has stabilized in order to facilitate recovery. Intrapleural analgesia has little to recommend it for rib fractures – it is laborious to perform, often results in a pneumothorax and is variable in its pattern of analgesia.

It is important to remember that rib fractures rarely exist in a vacuum and that the majority of patients will have associated injuries (e.g. pulmonary, cardiac, great vessels, spleen, liver). It is critical to ensure that the patient is euvolemic, stable and not in danger of decompensating prior to performing regional blockade, as the resultant sympathectomy may cause cardiovascular collapse.

Table 7.1 Analgesic modalities for rib fractures.

Analgesic modality	Advantages	Disadvantages
Systemic analgesia (NSAIDs, acetaminophen, opioids)	Easy to administer Can be titrated to various pain levels No risk of pneumothorax, dural puncture, LAST	Possible contraindication to NSAIDs if bleeding risk Respiratory depression and sedation from opioids
Thoracic epidural analgesia	Easy to perform, frequently performed (nursing familiarity) Excellent analgesia Ideal for bilateral rib fractures Little risk of LAST	Arterial hypotension common due to sympathectomy Conflict with some anticoagulation regimens Should not be performed in unconscious patients
Paravertebral nerve block	Excellent unilateral analgesia Technically easy No palpation of ribs required Can be done in presence of anticoagulation or in unconscious patients safely Hypotension/sympathectomy rare Can be done as catheter technique (one injection)	Small risk of pneumothorax Small risk of epidural spread Must be careful with dosages re: LAST (rapid absorption)
Intercostal nerve block	Excellent segmental analgesia Technically easy	Usually require multiple injections Palpation required (=pain) Only lasts 6–8 hours Risk of pneumothorax (1.5% per nerve blocked) Higher risk of LAST – ↑absorption from intercostal vessels
Intrapleural block	Can be moderately effective	Effectiveness variable; position-/gravity-dependent Technically challenging if not using chest tube for insertion High risk of LAST – large surface area Risk of lung parenchymal puncture

LAST, Local anesthetic systemic toxicity.

Which of the above techniques can be performed while the patient is receiving venous thrombosis prophylaxis?

All of the regional techniques can be employed effectively and safely, depending on the thromboprophylactic agent. One exception is TEA when twice-daily low molecular weight heparin is used, as the presence of an indwelling catheter is not recommended (see ASRA guidelines in Further reading in Horlocker *et al.* (2010)). Paravertebral blockade is an attractive choice in patients who are anticoagulated or on drugs that preclude epidural analgesia, as the risk of serious bleeding is very low.

You decide to perform intercostal blocks in the emergency room for pain relief, as the patient is clearly uncomfortable and is splinting when she breathes. The SpO$_2$ is still in the low 90s on facemask oxygen.

What are the technical considerations in performing ultrasound-guided intercostal blocks?

Thoracic spinal nerves exit the intervertebral foraminae and pass into the space between the innermost and internal intercostal muscles, where they remain for much of the remainder of their course (Figure 7.1). The classic description of each intercostal nerve traveling in the subcostal groove is outdated; anatomic studies have shown the actual position relative to the ribs to be quite variable. At the midaxillary line, the intercostal nerve gives rise to the lateral cutaneous branch, which pierces the internal and external intercostal muscles and supplies the muscles and skin of the lateral trunk. The continuation of the intercostal nerve terminates as the anterior cutaneous branch, which supplies the skin and muscles of the anterior trunk, including skin overlying the sternum and rectus abdominis.

Intercostal blockade results in ipsilateral analgesia. In contrast to paravertebral blockade, longitudinal spread to adjacent levels is less likely, although possible, especially with large volumes of injectate and/or injection sites close to the midline of the back. This block can be performed in the sitting, lateral decubitus or prone positions. Palpation of the inferior angle of the scapula allows for identification of the T7 vertebra and desired ribs to be blocked (Figure 7.2).

After sterile preparation, a linear ultrasound transducer is placed in the parasagittal orientation approximately 6–8 cm from the midline over the first rib to be blocked. The rib will be visualized as a hyperechoic convex linear density with deeper pleura on either side (Figure 7.3). Sliding the probe 1–2 cm inferiorly will center the probe over the intercostal space. The external intercostal muscle can be seen overlying the pleura; the nerve and vessels are not easily seen. A 50-mm short bevel needle is then inserted out-of-plane until tissue distortion is appreciated in the serratus anterior muscle overlying the ribs or the external intercostal muscle. At this point it is essential to hydrodissect with small (e.g. 0.5 ml) boluses of injectate down to the internal intercostal membrane. Passage through the membrane may not be appreciated by feel, but the subsequent bolus will be seen "pushing" the pleura down as injectate fills the space where the nerve and vessels lie. Prior to each bolus, aspiration for blood and/or air should be performed.

After 3–5 ml are deposited, the needle is withdrawn, the probe slid to the next desired level and the process repeated. A long-acting local anesthetic such as ropivacaine, bupivacaine or levobupivacaine 0.1–0.25% is the ideal choice. High concentrations are unnecessary and may lead to systemic toxicity owing to high absorption rates in this area.

The patient feels better immediately and is transferred to the trauma ICU. Six hours later, the nurse calls to say that the pain has returned. After examining and speaking with the patient, you decide to place a paravertebral catheter for long-acting pain control.

What are the technical considerations for inserting a paravertebral catheter?

The thoracic paravertebral space is a wedge-shaped area formed by the parietal pleura anterolaterally, the vertebral body, intervertebral disk and intervertebral foramen medially, and the superior costotransverse ligament posteriorly. The thoracic paravertebral space is continuous with the intercostal space laterally and the epidural space medially. In addition, with sufficient volume, spread occurs longitudinally both cranially and caudally.

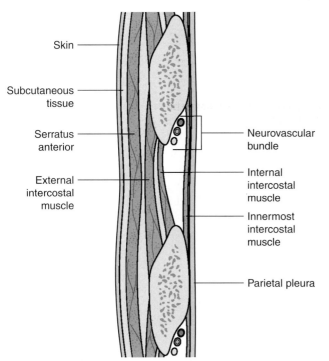

Figure 7.1 Parasagittal section of the posterolateral chest wall showing the relationship between the ribs, muscles and neurovascular structures.

Skin

Subcutaneous tissue

Serratus anterior

External intercostal muscle

Neurovascular bundle

Internal intercostal muscle

Innermost intercostal muscle

Parietal pleura

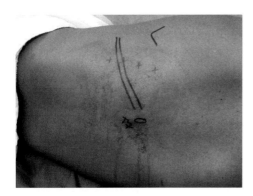

Figure 7.2 Positioning and landmarking for intercostal blocks. The T7 spinous process has been identified using the angle of the scapula, and the 7th rib marked. Each "X" marks a rib level to be blocked (T5–8 in this case).

The patient is positioned in the sitting or lateral decubitus position. The tips of the spinous processes corresponding to the fractured ribs should be drawn on the skin with a marker, using the angle of the scapula (T7) and the vertebra prominens (C7) as landmarks. The needle insertion site is marked on the skin 2.5 cm from the superior aspect of the spinous process corresponding to the middle of the desired block level, T6 or 7 in this patient (Figure 7.4).

After local skin infiltration, a 17-GA Tuohy needle is advanced perpendicularly to the skin. Constant attention to the depth of needle insertion and the medial–lateral needle

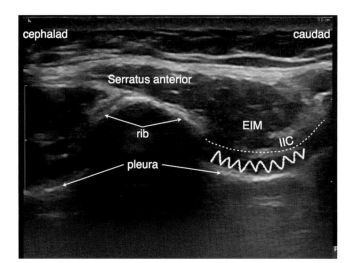

Figure 7.3 Sonoanatomy for intercostal blocks. The rib and pleura are both hyperechoic, and alternate as shallow and deep structures respectively. The target for needle tip advancement is between the internal intercostal membrane (IIC) and the parietal pleura, a space marked with the thick line. EIM, External intercostal muscle.

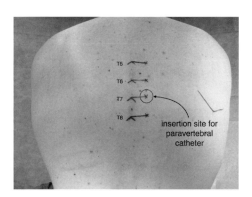

Figure 7.4 Landmarks for paravertebral block. Spinous processes for the desired levels are identified and points marked 2.5 cm lateral to their superior aspect. Single injections can be made at all levels to provide temporary relief. For a continuous catheter technique, the catheter should be placed at a midlevel point (T7 in this case).

orientation is critical to avoid complications. The transverse process should be contacted at a depth of 2–4 cm. If it is not, it is possible that the needle tip is lying between the transverse processes. In this case, further advancement could result in inadvertent deep insertion and possible pleural puncture. The needle should be withdrawn and redirected superiorly or inferiorly until bony contact is made at this depth.

After the transverse process is contacted, the needle is withdrawn to skin level and redirected 10° inferiorly to "walk off" the transverse process exactly 1 cm (Figures 7.5 and 7.6). To ensure the correct distance, once the transverse process is contacted, the needle should be regripped 1 cm away from the skin so that only a 1-cm deeper insertion can be made before skin contact with the fingers prevents further advancement.

The stylet is then removed and aspiration performed to rule out intravascular or intra-thoracic needle tip placement. A syringe containing local anesthetic is attached and 8–10 ml injected slowly (forceful injection can result in bilateral spread). The catheter can then be gently inserted to no more than 3 cm past the needle tip. The needle is withdrawn and

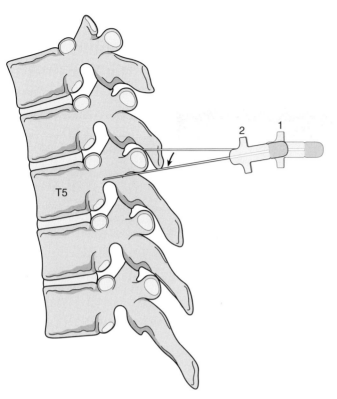

Figure 7.5 Needling sequence for paravertebral blockade. Step 1: the needle tip contacts the transverse process. Step 2: the needle is withdrawn, redirected 10° inferiorly and advanced 1 cm to lie beyond the transverse process.

the catheter secured to the skin. A further 8–10 ml is administered via the catheter, which should result in blockade of four to five dermatomes.

A long-acting local anesthetic such as ropivacaine, bupivacaine or levobupivacaine 0.1–0.25% is the ideal choice for this indication. Local anesthetic is infused at 10 ml/h or 6 ml/h when a patient-controlled regional dose (4 ml every 30 minutes) is planned.

Two hours later the ICU nurse calls you urgently, stating that the patient has developed sinus tachycardia (HR 115–120 bpm), hypotension (SBP 80 mmHg) and is disoriented.

What is your differential diagnosis?

Given the scenario, the differential should include tension pneumothorax, blunt cardiac injury/tamponade and LAST as the primary events to rule out. Other possibilities to rule out quickly include myocardial ischemia, anaphylaxis, pulmonary embolism and inadvertent drug administration.

You instruct the nurse to open the IV wide open and call for assistance. As you arrive at the bedside, the patient begins to have a tonic–clonic seizure. You now strongly suspect LAST as the problem.

How does local anesthetic systemic toxicity present?

The "classic" description involves subtle neurologic symptoms progressing to seizures, loss of consciousness, followed by cardiovascular manifestations. However, many cases present

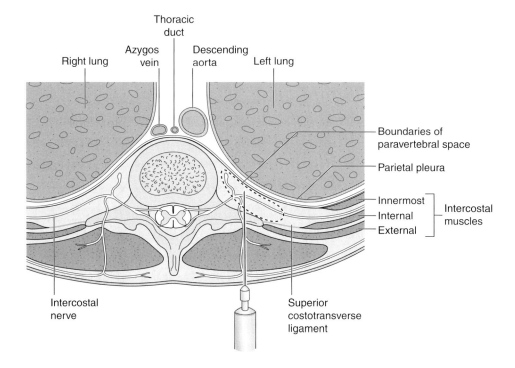

Figure 7.6 The paravertebral space (dotted line) and related structures. The needle tip is approximately 1 cm past the posterior surface of the transverse process.

initially with cardiovascular signs (11%) or a combination of neurologic symptoms and cardiovascular signs (44%).

1. Neurologic symptoms
   - Seizure (68%)
   - Agitation (11%)
   - Loss of consciousness (7%)
   - Dysarthria, perioral numbness, tinnitus, dizziness, dysphoria (18%)
2. Cardiovascular signs
   - Bradycardia/asystole (27%)
   - Hypotension (18%)
   - Tachycardia (16%)
   - VF/VT (13%)
   - Widening of QRS complex (12%)
   - ST changes, chest pain, dyspnea, hypertension (9%)
   - Ventricular ectopy (5%).

How is local anesthetic systemic toxicity treated?

1. Stop injecting local anesthetic.
2. Call for help.
3. Ensure adequate oxygenation and ventilation:
   - Mask ventilation ± endotracheal intubation
   - Critical in preventing hypoxia and acidosis, both of which potentiate local anesthetic toxicity.
4. Halt seizures:
   - Benzodiazepines are first-line treatment, e.g. midazolam 2–4 mg
   - Small doses of propofol (20–40 mg) are acceptable.
5. Circulatory support
   - IV crystalloid
   - Cardiopulmonary resuscitation/advanced cardiac life support (CPR/ACLS) if severe hypotension/pulseless
   - Vasopressor therapy is controversial based on a number of experimental studies. If cardiac arrest occurs, epinephrine should be used in small doses (10–100 mcg)
   - Do not use vasopressin, calcium channel blockers, β-blockers or lidocaine in treatment of cardiac arrest/arrhythmias
   - Amiodarone is antiarrhythmic of choice.
6. Lipid emulsion therapy
   - Consider administering at the first sign of toxicity (even mild symptoms)
   - Dosing regimen
     - 1.5 ml/kg of 20% lipid emulsion bolus (approximately 100 ml for most adults)
     - Infusion of 0.25 ml/kg/min, continued for at least 10 minutes after return of circulatory stability
     - If required, re-bolus and increase infusion dose to 0.5 ml/kg/min
     - Maximum dose = 10 ml/kg over first 30 minutes
   - Propofol is not indicated. While it has a lipid as a constituent, the amount required to achieve an effect would cause profound circulatory depression.
7. Consider institution of cardiopulmonary bypass (if available) and resuscitation if not responsive to the above measures.

Further reading

Cohn, S. M., Dubose, J. J. (2010). Pulmonary contusion: an update on recent advances in clinical management. *World Journal of Surgery*, **34**, 1959–70.

de Moya, M. A., Manolakaki, D., Chang, Y. *et al.* (2011). Blunt pulmonary contusion: admission computed tomography scan predicts mechanical ventilation. *The Journal of Trauma*, **71**, 1543–7.

Di Gregorio, G., Neal, J. M., Rosenquist, R. W., Weinberg, G. L. (2010). Clinical presentation of local anesthetic systemic toxicity: a review of published cases, 1979 to 2009. *Regional Anesthesia and Pain Medicine*, **35**, 181–7.

Dravid, R. M., Paul, R. E. (2007). Interpleural block – part 1. *Anaesthesia*, **62**, 1039–49.

Horlocker, T. T., Wedel, D. J., Rowlingson, J. C. *et al.* (2010). Regional anesthesia in the patient receiving antithrombotic or thrombolytic therapy: American Society of Regional Anesthesia and Pain Medicine Evidence-Based Guidelines. 3rd edn. *Regional Anesthesia and Pain Medicine*, **35**, 64–101.

Livingston, D. H., Shogan, B., John, P., Lavery, R. F. (2008). CT diagnosis of rib fractures and the prediction of acute respiratory failure. *The Journal of Trauma*, **64**, 905–11.

Mohta, M., Verma, P., Saxena, A. K. *et al.* (2009). Prospective, randomized comparison of continuous thoracic epidural and thoracic paravertebral infusion in patients with unilateral multiple fractured ribs – a pilot study. *The Journal of Trauma*, **66**, 1096–101.

Shanti, C. M., Carlin, A. M., Tyburski, J. G. (2001). Incidence of pneumothorax from intercostal nerve block for analgesia in rib fractures. *The Journal of Trauma*, **51**, 536–9.

Sharma, O. P., Oswanski, M. F., Jolly, S. *et al.* (2008). Perils of rib fractures. *The American Surgeon*, **74**, 310–14.

Regional anesthesia, trauma and complex regional pain syndrome

Key aspects of case

1. Geriatric considerations for trauma.

2. Considerations for upper limb brachial plexus blockade and chronic obstructive pulmonary disease (COPD).

3. Prevention of the progression of acute pain to complex regional pain syndrome (CRPS).

Case presentation

A 76-year-old woman presents to hospital after suffering a fall on an icy sidewalk. She was able to break her fall with her outstretched arm, and is now complaining of pain in her right wrist; examination and radiography reveal a displaced distal radius fracture. There are no other injuries apart from some soft-tissue bruising on her lower extremities. She has a 60 pack-year history of smoking and takes inhaled steroids and beta-agonists for emphysema, for which she is admitted once or twice per year for acute exacerbations. Her breathing feels fine today and she has not had a recent flare-up. The orthopedic surgeon plans to perform an open reduction and internal fixation of her fracture later today.

Case discussion

What is different about the nature of geriatric trauma?

The elderly patient (commonly defined as age >65 years) presents a unique challenge to trauma care providers owing to the age-related decrease in physiologic reserve and increase in comorbidities. Increasing age is associated with increased mortality, independent of injury severity score (ISS) or GCS, and trauma represents the seventh leading cause of death in geriatric adults in the USA and the fifth leading cause of death in elderly Canadians.

The epidemiology of trauma in this population is different than in younger adults, with falls accounting for the vast majority (40–72%) of injuries. Motor vehicle accidents, the number one cause of trauma in younger adults, still make up a large proportion (approximately 25%) of injury mechanisms. Burns are also more frequent in this cohort, perhaps because of impaired hearing or vision, or increased reaction time. Mortality more frequently occurs later in the hospital course for older adults (versus prehospital for younger adults) because of the lower energy nature of geriatric trauma in general.

Table 8.1 Considerations during the primary survey of geriatric trauma

Element of primary survey	Considerations
Airway	Dentition may be poor or artificial Arthritis of the neck and temporomandibular junction (especially rheumatoid arthritis) may make intubation challenging Reduce dose of sedative/hypnotic for intubation because of ↓cardiovascular reserve
Breathing	Oxygenation is crucial; do not withhold O_2 for patients with COPD Chest wall is less elastic→higher rate of rib fractures, pulmonary contusion and blunt myocardial injury
Circulation	Pre-existing hypertension may mask hypovolemia in face of "normal" blood pressure Responsiveness to catecholamines *and* autonomic reflexes are blunted→may not develop tachycardia May be on beta-blockers, which may mask cardiovascular responses
Disability	Prone to confusion→difficulty in interpreting GCS Vertebral osteoporosis and spinal stenosis→increased risk for cord injury
Exposure and environment	Thin skin increases risk for hypothermia

Common injuries include fractures of the rib, sternum, vertebrae, hip and distal forearm, owing to a high prevalance of osteoporosis.

What special considerations should be taken into account in the primary survey?

While the initial injury assessment and resuscitation of the geriatric patient is essentially the same as for young adults, it is important to bear in mind some of the anatomic and physiologic differences that may impact management (Table 8.1).

What are the options for analgesia for the patient's broken radius?

Systemic analgesia with opioids is an option but has the downside of respiratory depression in a patient who is already at high risk for pulmonary compromise. In addition, opioids tend to worsen delirium in elderly adults. NSAIDs are good analgesics, but discussion should take place with the orthopedic team regarding the risk for osteoblast inhibition.

Regional analgesic options include brachial plexus block and selective distal blocks of the forearm (see Chapter 12). The advantages of brachial plexus block include a rapid onset of dense, complete analgesia of the wrist and the avoidance of any systemic medications that might alter sensorium or impact the respiratory system (i.e. opioids). Brachial plexus block is generally well tolerated, but consideration should be given in this patient to the effect of the block on pulmonary function caused by any inadvertent blockade of the phrenic nerve.

To what extent does brachial plexus block result in phrenic nerve blockade?

The incidence of phrenic nerve blockade appears to be related to block location and dose of local anesthetic. Early studies demonstrated that 100% of patients receiving an interscalene block (ISB) developed hemidiaphragmatic paralysis, although the volume of local anesthetic was relatively high (up to 52 ml). More recent studies of ISB with reduced doses have shown a reduction in this side effect. Ultrasound-guided ISB performed using 5 ml of ropivacaine leads to an incidence of phrenic blockade of 33–50% compared to 60% with 10 ml and 100% with 20 ml; analgesic effect with any of these doses appears to be similar.

The more distal the block is performed on the brachial plexus, the lower the likelihood of phrenic nerve blockade. Supraclavicular block may still carry an incidence of 0–60%, whereas the axillary approach is free from this side effect. The infraclavicular approach is largely thought not to impact the phrenic nerve, although there are scattered case reports of this occurring, perhaps related to anatomical variants or large doses used.

What impact does hemidiaphragmatic paralysis have on pulmonary function?

In the healthy patient, hemidiaphragmatic paralysis leads to a 25–30% decrease in both the forced vital capacity (FVC) and the forced expiratory volume over 1 second (FEV_1). These reductions in flow are typically well tolerated both in healthy patients and those with obstructive airways disease such as asthma, emphysema and chronic bronchitis. Patients occasionally report dyspnea following ISB with resultant phrenic nerve blockade, but this is easily treated in most cases with reassurance, and an explanation that this is a frequent side effect that will disappear when the block wears off.

Careful consideration should be made when planning brachial plexus blockade in patients with severe pulmonary disease. As stated above, patients with obstructive disease do well in general, especially emphysematous patients in whom the hemidiaphragm is already almost maximally flattened. Patients that are dependent on intact diaphragmatic excursion (e.g. those with ankylosing spondylitis, neuromuscular disease or some restrictive lung diseases) will be most adversely affected by phrenic nerve paralysis. In this group, a distal approach (such as infraclavicular or axillary) should be considered.

What are the advantages and disadvantages of placing a continuous brachial plexus catheter in this patient?

Advantages to a continuous technique include the ability to provide prolonged analgesia throughout her treatment and recovery phases. The principal benefit is a substantial reduction in the need for opioid analgesia, and the side effects thereof, namely respiratory depression, constipation, delirium and dysphoria.

One disadvantage to a continuous block is the potential difficulty in neurologic assessment of the wrist and hand, although this can be overcome by stopping the infusion, allowing sensory and motor recovery, followed by reinitiation of the block afterwards. A proximal approach, such as interscalene or supraclavicular, is probably best avoided in this patient, as continual blockade of the phrenic nerve may result in atelectasis, hypoxemia and respiratory distress that can be avoided with a more distal approach.

You decide to place an ultrasound-guided continuous axillary catheter. What are the technical considerations for this technique?

Axillary catheters can be tricky for several reasons. First, the neurovascular structures are quite superficial and it is easy to puncture a vein with a large, blunt catheter insertion needle, especially because just a small amount of pressure applied to the skin from the ultrasound probe tends to collapse the veins on the sonographic image. Second, the skin is quite mobile here, and securing the catheter so that it does not become displaced is challenging.

The patient's arm should be abducted gently to 90° and the axillary area thoroughly disinfected. The ultrasound transducer is placed on the arm just distal to the insertion of the pectoralis major muscle (Figure 8.1). The first landmark is the axillary artery, which, with the help of the color Doppler function, should be readily apparent (Figure 8.2). It is useful to gently release the pressure on the transducer to reveal any veins that had been collapsed.

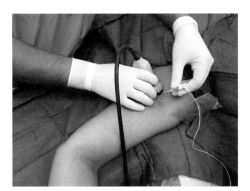

Figure 8.1 Transducer and needle position for ultrasound-guided axillary brachial plexus block.

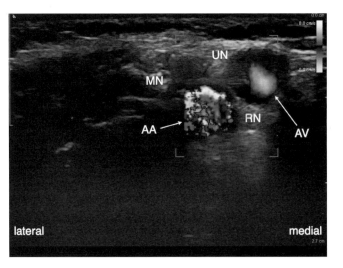

Figure 8.2 Sonoanatomy of the axilla highlighting vascular structures. The axillary artery (AA) and vein (AV) are easily identified with the use of color Doppler. MN, Median nerve; RN, radial nerve; UN, ulnar nerve.

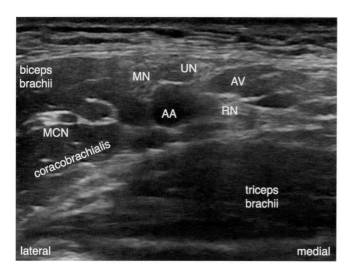

Figure 8.3 Sonoanatomy of the axilla. AA, Axillary artery; AV, axillary vein; MCN, musculocutaneous nerve; MN, median nerve; RN, radial nerve; UN, ulnar nerve.

The median, ulnar and radial nerves are clustered around the axillary artery, often at 11 o'clock, 2 o'clock and 5 o'clock, respectively (Figure 8.3). However, with a catheter technique it is ultimately less important to see each individual nerve than it is to place the catheter tip, and hence the local anesthetic, adjacent to the artery.

The needle can be inserted either in-plane from the lateral (superior) aspect, or out-of-plane. This decision is occasionally made on the basis of where the veins lie with respect to the projected needle path. However, one advantage to the in-plane approach is that the catheter can be tunneled subcutaneously for several centimeters prior to arriving at the target. The needle is advanced gently until the tip is visualized immediately adjacent to the artery (in our institution, we usually attempt to put the tip at about 6–7 o'clock). After negative aspiration, 2–3 ml of local anesthetic are injected to ensure proper location. The catheter is then advanced slowly, *but no more than 2–3 cm beyond the tip of the needle*. Further insertion only increases the risk of malposition, failed block and intravascular catheter placement. Once the needle is withdrawn, the catheter is aspirated again and a further 2–3 ml of local anesthetic bolused while observing for appropriate spread. Frequently the catheter has to be withdrawn 1–1.5 cm. Once in the correct position (i.e. adjacent to the artery), additional local anesthetic can be administered up to a total of 15–20 ml.

For surgical anesthesia, we often choose a local anesthetic such as mepivacaine 1.5% or lidocaine 2% to provide rapid, dense anesthesia. Postoperatively, the patient should receive a continuous infusion of a low concentration local anesthetic (e.g. ropivacaine 0.2%) at 5–8 ml/h, with the option of a bolus dose of 5 ml every 30–60 minutes.

Catheter securement is challenging in the axilla because of skin laxity on arm movement. For this reason, the following method is recommended to secure axillary catheters.

1. Dry the area carefully with gauze (do not pull out the catheter!).

2. If the out-of-plane approach was used, it is useful to tunnel the catheter subcutaneously in a superolateral direction. Insert the Tuohy catheter needle under the skin, starting at a point over the anterior deltoid muscle, and emerge immediately adjacent to the catheter. Insert the free end of the catheter through the needle in a retrograde fashion; once it emerges at the hub, feed most of the remainder of the catheter through, then remove the

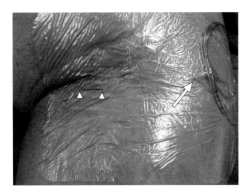

Figure 8.4 Catheter securing technique for continuous axillary blocks. The initial portion of catheter emerging from the skin (arrowheads) is tunnelled under the skin for several centimeters, emerging over the anterior deltoid muscle (arrow) where it can be coiled and taped in place in an attempt to decrease the risk of displacement.

needle carefully. Pull the remaining catheter so that a small "bridge" lies on the skin (Figure 8.4).

3. Apply Dermabond to all the skin/catheter sites and wait for it to polymerize (60 s).
4. Apply sterile transparent dressings (e.g. Tegaderm™).

What is the incidence of CRPS following distal forearm fractures?

Wrist fractures are particularly prone to the development of CRPS. Up to 25–30% of Colles' fractures are felt to have some element of CRPS as early as 1 week after injury, including finger tenderness, swelling, finger stiffness and vasomotor instability. Severity can vary from very mild to incapacitating, and can last for decades. Every effort possible should be made to reduce the likelihood of this adverse outcome from developing.

What interventions can be employed to reduce the risk of development of CRPS?

This is a controversial area, and there is scant literature supporting many of the interventions that have been attempted to reduce this complication (e.g. mannitol, calcitonin, corticosteroids, gabapentinoids). Regional anesthetic blocks have the theoretical advantage of halting the sympathetic efferent flow to the extremity, which has been implicated in CRPS type I. There are reports of patients with a prior history of CRPS who have subsequently had their disease "rekindled" following general anesthesia alone, suggesting that unimpeded sympathetic reflex arcs are at least partially responsible for this sympathetically mediated pain syndrome. Others have reported cases of serial orthopedic operations in patients with a history of CRPS; following general anesthesia, the dystrophy returned, but after peripheral nerve block or intravenous regional anesthesia, the disease remained quiescent. This lends support to the idea that sympathectomy helps to prevent CRPS following surgery. However, while this is an attractive theory, large-scale randomized controlled studies are lacking.

If a block is to be performed, logic dictates that the patient will get the most benefit in terms of risk reduction with a continuous technique. If a single-injection block is used, the benefit is only conferred for the duration of the block, and 12–24 hours later the barrage of sympathetic impulses will start up again.

The only intervention that has been shown in a randomized controlled fashion to reduce the incidence of CRPS after surgery for wrist or ankle fracture is vitamin C. A dose of 500–1000 mg PO daily for 45–50 days has been shown to reduce the risk significantly, from approximately 10% to 2%.

Further reading

Besse, J.-L., Gadeyne, S., Galand-Desmé, S., Lerat, J.-L., Moyen, B. (2009). Effect of vitamin C on prevention of complex regional pain syndrome type I in foot and ankle surgery. *Foot and Ankle Surgery: Official Journal of the European Society of Foot and Ankle Surgeons*, **15**, 179–82.

da Costa, V. V., de Oliveira, S. B., Fernandes, M. do C. B., Saraiva, R. Â. (2011). Incidence of regional pain syndrome after carpal tunnel release. Is there a correlation with the anesthetic technique? *Revista Brasileira De Anestesiologia*, **61**, 425–33.

Jenson, M. G., Sorensen, R. F. (2006). Early use of regional and local anesthesia in a combat environment may prevent the development of complex regional pain syndrome in wounded combatants. *Military Medicine*, **171**, 396–8.

Lee, J.-H., Cho, S.-H., Kim, S.-H. *et al.* (2011). Ropivacaine for ultrasound-guided interscalene block: 5 mL provides similar analgesia but less phrenic nerve paralysis than 10 mL. *Canadian Journal of Anaesthesia*, **58**, 1001–6.

Lewis, M. C., Abouelenin, K., Paniagua, M. (2007). Geriatric trauma: special considerations in the anesthetic management of the injured elderly patient. *Anesthesiology Clinics*, **25**, 75–90.

Riazi, S., Carmichael, N., Awad, I., Holtby, R. M., McCartney, C. J. L. (2008). Effect of local anaesthetic volume (20 vs 5 ml) on the efficacy and respiratory consequences of ultrasound-guided interscalene brachial plexus block. *British Journal of Anaesthesia*, **101**, 549–56.

Rocco, A. G. (1993). Sympathetically maintained pain may be rekindled by surgery under general anesthesia. *Anesthesiology*, **79**, 865.

Viel, E. J., Pelissier, J., Eledjam, J. J. (1994). Sympathetically maintained pain after surgery may be prevented by regional anesthesia. *Anesthesiology*, **81**, 265–6.

Zollinger, P. E., Tuinebreijer, W. E., Breederveld, R. S., Kreis, R. W. (2007). Can vitamin C prevent complex regional pain syndrome in patients with wrist fractures? A randomized, controlled, multicenter dose-response study. *The Journal of Bone and Joint Surgery. American Volume*, **89**, 1424–31.

Regional anesthesia and combat care

Key aspects of case

1. Unique considerations for military trauma.
2. Role of regional analgesia for initial pain management and facilitation of airborne transport to advanced care facilities.

Case presentation

A 20-year-old army private stationed in Afghanistan is traveling along a remote road in a light-armored vehicle as part of a convoy when an improvised explosive device (IED) detonates nearby, overturning the vehicle. He is wearing body armor and a helmet, but is knocked unconscious by the blast. He awakens minutes later on the road, while being attended to by another soldier. His injuries include a complete amputation of his left leg at the mid-tibia and a severe crush injury to his left hand. He is having trouble breathing and is given IV morphine as he is loaded on an ambulance for transfer to a level II facility.

Case discussion

What are the general differences between the management of military versus civilian trauma?

While many specifics about the management of wounded soldiers and civilians are different, the management of the exsanguinating patient should not vary. Most of the advances in the treatment of civilian trauma worldwide have come as a result of experience in war-time. For example, the concept of damage control resuscitation and the early use of plasma and packed red blood cells for resuscitation in place of crystalloid that is used today was largely developed by military physicians. Some differences include:

- The frequent occurrence of large numbers of patients presenting at once for emergent care
- The need to provide care in austere and often hostile ("under fire") conditions
- A relative lack of providers compared with civilian practice
- A relative shortage of advanced or scarce resources (e.g. CT scanners, operating rooms, blood)
- The means by which to transfer patients to the next level of care (i.e. ambulances) may not be available.

Table 9.1 Typical findings resulting from primary blast injury

Injury	Findings
Pulmonary contusion	Crackles ↓Breath sounds, dullness to percussion Dyspnea, hypoxemia Hemoptysis Chest pain
Pulmonary laceration/pneumothorax/hemothorax	Hyperresonance, ↓breath sounds Subcutaneous emphysema Hemoptysis Hypotension Hypoxemia
Gastrointestinal tract	Edema, hemorrhage, rupture Absent bowel sounds Abdominal pain Bright red blood per rectum Nausea/vomiting
Auditory system	Tympanic membrane rupture Sensorineural or conductive hearing loss

For these reasons, the concept of triaging is extremely important in military medicine: this is the judicious use of limited resources to help the largest number of patients.

What is the pattern of trauma with blast injury?

Since World War II, there has been a relative decrease in lower extremity and torso injuries, and an increase in head, neck and upper extremity injuries. This is related to two factors: improvements in body armor design and the increased use of IEDs. Primary blast injury refers to the tissue injury that results from the pressure wave generated that can reach up to 2100 kph (1300 mph). The organs that are principally affected are those that contain tissue/gas interfaces, such as the pulmonary, gastrointestinal and auditory organs (Table 9.1). There is often an absence of external injuries associated with primary blast injury, which makes these potentially lethal injuries easy to overlook, and a thorough evaluation to rule out and treat is warranted.

In contrast, secondary blast injuries are caused by objects such as shrapnel from the explosion striking and/or penetrating the body. Many IEDs are designed to generate shrapnel (e.g. nail bombs). Tertiary blast injury refers to the body being thrown against stationary objects such as buildings, and these are typically characterized by severe fractures. Other injuries that are common as a result of explosions are burns, amputations and crush injuries.

How is medical support during military engagements organized?

Another trend in military medicine that has led to improved outcomes in the past several decades has been the emphasis on improving far-forward care and ensuring the timely evacuation of casualties in a continuous chain of care.

The USA and UK are examples of nations that provide tiered medical support to their troops, starting at the geographic site of injury and moving through increasingly sophisticated levels until reaching definitive care hospitals in the home country following repatriation (Figure 9.1).

On the battlefield (level I), soldiers are provided with initial care by medics or "buddy first aid" by other soldiers. In general, military personnel are trained in the use of one-hand tourniquets and in basic wound dressings. Following initial first aid, casualties are transferred to a nearby battalion aid station, where they are triaged by a physician or physician's assistant as to the necessity for further escalation of evacuation. Those that require such are transferred by ground ambulance or helicopter to a level II facility, often located on a forward operating base (these are typically staffed with emergency physicians and nurses), before being triaged and transferred to a level III facility, which is a hospital on a main base of operations. These facilities have the capability to provide advanced orthopedic, neurosurgical and critical care recovery before the patient is flown via fixed-wing aircraft out of the theater of operations to a hospital in the home country (level IV), where they can receive definitive surgical care and rehabilitation. The US military has an intermediate stop in Landstuhl, Germany, where a full-service hospital is available at their base. The care of US soldiers at hospitals within the USA can therefore be considered level V.

Forward surgical teams are small (20-member) teams of surgeons, anesthetists and nurses and logisticians that can be deployed quickly in situations where casualties may not

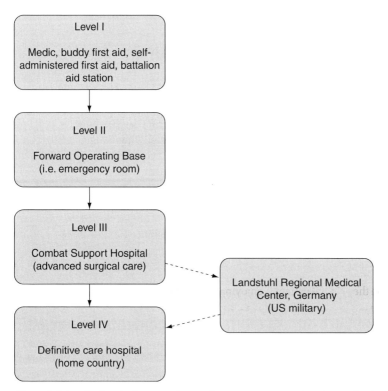

Figure 9.1 Levels of medical support during military operations. Levels I–III are in the theater of operations, whereas level IV (or V) are located in the home (or ally) nation.

survive transfer to a level III facility. They have the ability to perform damage control surgery and treat life-threatening traumatic injuries before continuing up the chain of facilities.

The patient is triaged, resuscitated and stabilized and finally transferred to the level III facility where he is taken to an operating room for irrigation, debridement and possible limb salvage of his hand. His GCS on arrival is 13, and he has had 18 mg of morphine intra-venously since his injury. He is wearing a semi-rigid cervical collar. His vitals are BP 108/78, HR 99, RR 22, SpO_2 96% on facemask O_2. His chest X-ray shows diffuse airspace disease of the left lung, and a well-positioned left-sided chest tube which was placed for a hemopneu-mothorax. He is otherwise healthy with no allergies. Point of care testing shows his hemoglobin to be 13 mg/dl.

What are your priorities for the anesthetic management of this patient?

- Prevent complications related to his traumatic brain injury: avoid hypoxemia, hypercarbia, hypotonic fluids; keep systolic blood pressure >90 mmHg
- Prevent further worsening of his respiratory status owing to presumed pulmonary contusion. Avoidance of pulmonary intubation and mechanical ventilation may prevent secondary pneumonia and other ventilator-associated complications
- Optimize the chances of successful limb salvage by preventing sympathetically mediated vasoconstriction in the left arm
- If possible and a safe alternative exists, avoid managing the airway in a patient with C-spine precautions and a presumed full stomach
- Provide quality and long-lasting analgesia for two severely painful extremity injuries that does not conflict with the above priorities.

The patient is cooperative and agrees to your plan of dual continuous perineural catheters. You expertly place both a left infraclavicular catheter and a left popliteal catheter and surgery commences uneventfully. No sedation is administered.

What are the specific advantages to using regional techniques as the primary anesthetic in this setting?

- **Freedom:** in an environment that is relatively resource-poor, the avoidance of general anesthesia liberates the anesthesiologist to tend to other matters. For example, in a mass casualty situation, his/her skills may be better put to use resuscitating or anesthetizing a second or third patient while the original patient is enjoying a stable and pain-free surgical experience.
- **Space:** the reduced length of stay associated with regional anesthesia and, in particular, peripheral nerve block (PNB) techniques allows these soldiers to be rapidly discharged from the field hospital and moved to the next echelon in their care, thereby creating more beds for the next round of casualties.
- **Safety:** compared with PNBs, general anesthesia in the fresh trauma patient is associated with an increased incidence of hypotension and hypothermia, and an increased risk of gastric aspiration.

The initial surgical procedure finishes and the patient states that he feels no pain in his injured extremities. In the recovery room he learns that he will be boarding an aeromedical transport plane to fly him back home to receive definitive care and rehabilitation.

What are the challenges in providing care during aeromedical transport?

- **Environment:** average ambient noise levels inside the cabin of a large transport plane can exceed 75 dB, and hearing protection is mandatory for all providers. This limits the value of auditory alarms, oximeter tones and other auditory cues and puts a greater emphasis on visual data. However, lighting can also be minimal, rendering the normal visual cues, such as cyanosis or the character of drainage fluid, less useful without portable sources of light. Finally, temperature is often kept low, and active warmers are required to prevent hypothermia.

- **Vibration:** during the majority of takeoffs in the theater of operations, the pilot of an evacuation transport will attempt to climb to an altitude of 8000 feet as quickly as possible, so as to minimize the threat from hostile forces. The reverse maneuver is often performed during landing. This places enormous strain on the airframe and the objects and people within it. Patients who are comfortable at rest often find their injuries very painful while in transport.

- **Altitude:** flying at a pressurized cabin altitude of 8000 feet for 10 or more hours may have a deleterious effect on a patient's wellbeing, especially if they have the potential for gas evolution, such as an untreated pneumothorax, pneumocephalus or air in or behind the globe. Similarly, the effect of lowered pressures on the size and tension within endotracheal tube and urinary catheter balloons must be taken into account. Hypoxemia is usually not an issue as oxygen is available, unless the patient is severely hypoxemic at baseline.

What are the advantages of peripheral nerve blocks in aeromedical transport?

Until the last decade, injured soldiers were treated with oral and occasional IV opioid for pain while in transport. However, unlike a civilian ICU, where 1:1 attention is provided at all times and interventions are provided on an as-needed basis, the practical aspects of military transport dictate that there are many periods of time where the patient has no access to IV or PO medication. For example, the transfer from hospital to ambulance, ambulance to plane, and the intervals during takeoff and landing that can last up to an hour are all periods where a patient relying solely on parenteral or oral analgesia might suffer. It has been reported that over 80% of American casualties transported from Iraq to Germany complained of uncontrolled pain defined on a numeric rating scale of >5.

Moreover, the pain associated with air transport itself can be excruciating, especially for amputation injuries where the stump is striking the litter or other piece of equipment with every jolt. The delayed analgesia afforded by IV or PO opioids is not well matched to this type of pain.

Continuous PNBs address this issue both simply and elegantly. Chief amongst their advantages are the following:

- Low cost
- Easy to administer: elastomeric pumps can last for several days and do not require electricity or any other adjunctive equipment
- Able to target the painful areas specifically without rendering the sensorium dulled
- Free from other opioid-related side effects such as sedation, nausea and vomiting, constipation, pruritus and immunosuppression
- Titratable: if breakthrough pain occurs with an increased intensity of pain stimulus (i.e. a rattly C-130 Hercules transport), the concentration of local anesthetic can be increased.

Perhaps more compelling is the ability to avoid the respiratory depression and sedation associated with opioids. This is particularly true in patients such as this one, where traumatic brain injury and pulmonary contusion put him at risk for increased intracranial pressure and respiratory distress with opioid use. Without continuous nerve blocks there is an increased likelihood that this patient would require endotracheal intubation and mechanical ventilation during transport.

Are there risks to long-term perineural catheterization?

The biggest fear in leaving catheters in place for more than 48 hours is the increased risk of infection, which has been shown in civilian trauma and elective orthopedic procedures, with a rate of approximately 0.1%. One report reviewed 287 veterans at Walter Reed Army Medical Center who had undergone continuous nerve catheter placement for a total of 1700 catheter-days. The infection rate was found to be 1.9%, but these were all superficial and resolved with removal of the catheter. The same group has commented that over 50 catheters have been placed in *battlefield conditions* (i.e. less than ideal sterility) and kept in place for 2–17 days with no infectious complications.

On the other hand, a recent case series from Brooke Army Medical Center in Texas reported that, of 300 catheters placed over a 3-year period, six resulted in infection (2%), but half of these were associated with deep tissue abscesses that required operations. The catheters were *in situ* for 4–11 days before diagnosis was made, prompting the authors to revise an institutional policy that now limits duration to only 5 days.

Clearly, a risk–benefit analysis must be made for each patient. The vast majority (>98%) of these young, otherwise healthy, soldiers appear to suffer no infectious complications. There may be other risk factors that predispose to abscesses – in the above report from Brooke Army Medical Center, all of the patients requiring surgery were instrumented with stimulating catheters, whereas non-stimulating catheter placement was associated with only superficial skin infection. The authors speculate that the metal coil in the center of the stimulating catheter could lead to microhematomas, a rich breeding ground for bacteria. This question remains unanswered.

Further reading

Buckenmaier, C. C., McKnight, G. M., Winkley, J. V. *et al.* (2005). Continuous peripheral nerve block for battlefield anesthesia and evacuation. *Regional Anesthesia and Pain Medicine*, **30**, 202–5.

Guzzi, L. M., Argyros, G. (1996). The management of blast injury. *European Journal of Emergency Medicine: Official Journal of the European Society for Emergency Medicine*, **3**, 252–5.

Hunter, J. G. (2010). Managing pain on the battlefield: an introduction to continuous peripheral nerve blocks. *Journal of the Royal Army Medical Corps*, **156**, 230–2.

Johannigman, J. A. (2008). Maintaining the continuum of en route care. *Critical Care Medicine*, **36**, S377–82.

Lai, T. T., Jaeger, L., Jones, B. L., Kaderbek, E. W., Malchow, R. J. (2011). Continuous peripheral nerve block catheter infections in combat-related injuries: a case report of five soldiers from Operation Enduring Freedom/Operation Iraqi Freedom. *Pain Medicine*, **12**, 1676–81.

Ling, G. S. F., Rhee, P., Ecklund, J. M. (2010). Surgical innovations arising from the Iraq and Afghanistan wars. *Annual Review of Medicine*, **61**, 457–68.

Stojadinovic, A., Auton, A., Peoples, G. E. *et al.* (2006). Responding to challenges in modern combat casualty care: innovative use of advanced regional anesthesia. *Pain Medicine*, **7**, 330–8.

Regional anesthesia for pediatric trauma

Key aspects of case

1. Unique considerations for pediatric trauma.
2. Assessment of pain in children.
3. Brachial plexus blockade in children.

Case presentation

A 6-year-old girl falls off her bicycle while riding on the street outside her home. She is taken to hospital by her parents and presents with complaints of pain in her right elbow and the right upper quadrant of her abdomen. Upon questioning, her mother tells you that the child came to a sudden stop after hitting the curb and, after striking the handlebars, landed directly on the ground on her right side, breaking her fall with her flexed arm. She did not hit her head, nor lose consciousness. The primary survey reveals no apparent life-threatening injuries. Her vitals are: HR 98 bpm, BP 95/47, RR 25 and temperature 36.8°C. Examination reveals a moderately distressed child with a swollen, bruised right elbow; neurovascular exam of her forearm and hand is normal. She has some minor scrapes on her chest, and her abdomen is tender to palpation on the right side. An elbow radiograph shows a slightly displaced supracondylar fracture. She is sent for an abdominal CT scan, which shows a 3-cm parenchymal tear of the liver with extravasation of IV contrast. No other abdominal injuries are noted.

Case discussion

What are the key differences between pediatric and adult trauma?

Trauma is the leading cause of death in children and young adults. Many of the common mechanisms are the same as in older adults, such as motor vehicle accidents and falls, but drowning and death from fire and burns are more prevalent in children than in adults. Sadly, child abuse is also a common cause of injury in the pediatric population, especially young children and infants.

Children have several anatomical differences that lead to distinct patterns of injury (Table 10.1). Head size is larger, leading to a higher incidence of traumatic brain injury. Children have less fat and connective tissue, and their organs are in closer proximity to each other and to the surface, leading to a higher frequency of multiple organ injuries.

Table 10.1 Typical patterns of injury in children based on mechanism of injury

Mechanism of injury	Typical patterns of injury
Fall from bicycle	Wrist/forearm/arm fractures Head/neck lacerations and fracture if no helmet Struck handlebars: abdominal wall and internal abdominal injuries
Fall from height	Low (e.g. from chair): upper extremity fractures, head and neck injuries High (e.g. from roof): upper and lower extremity fractures, head and neck injuries, thoracic/pelvic injuries
Struck by motor vehicle	Low speed: lower extremity fractures High speed: multiple trauma Backed over by vehicle: closed head injury, torso trauma, upper and lower extremity, death
Passenger in motor vehicle collision	Wearing seat belt: chest/abdomen injuries, lumbar spine fracture Unrestrained: multiple trauma, head and neck injuries, death

The skeleton of a child is incompletely ossified, and bones are more flexible. For this reason, blunt thoracic trauma should prompt a thorough investigation for possible soft organ damage despite an absence of overlying rib fractures (as might be seen in an adult). Children are also more prone to the effects of hypothermia owing to a larger surface area: mass ratio.

Does the liver injury require operative management?

Current practice for blunt abdominal trauma resulting in isolated hepatic injury is typically non-operative, providing the patient is hemodynamically stable. More routine use of early CT scanning in the trauma workup has led to a decrease in the rate of laparotomies and laparoscopies for liver injury, and also facilitates specific characterization of the injury (e.g. location, depth, associated degree of hemoperitoneum, etc.). The patient should be monitored carefully for changes in hemodynamic status, and repeat hemoglobin levels should be assessed to guide transfusion therapy and the possible need for operative management if hemostasis is not achieved.

The patient is crying and is cradling her injured arm. She appears to be in a moderate amount of discomfort.

How is pain assessed in children?

Pain is often poorly treated in children because of an underestimation of the intensity of pain and the fear of risk of complications from analgesics such as opioids. The ability to express subjective pain is largely dependent on cognitive and language ability. For small children and infants, non-verbal signs play a large role in the assessment, and these behaviors have been well characterized and validated. For example, the neonatal infant pain scale assigns values to each of the following to develop a composite score: facial expression, cry, breathing, arm and leg movements, and alertness. Older children that can understand questions and verbalize pain are able to use pain assessment tools such as the FACES pain scale (Figure 10.1). This valid and reliable tool is recommended for children across the age ranges of 4–16 years,

Figure 10.1 FACES pain scale tool for the assessment of pediatric pain. Children are asked to indicate "how much they hurt," and a numerical value (0, 2, 4, 6, 8 or 10) is assigned, which permits longitudinal evaluation. The FACES pain scale has been reproduced with permission of the International Association for the Study of Pain® (IASP®). The scale may not be reproduced for any other purpose without permission.

and is simple to use. Patients are instructed as to what each facial depiction means, and then asked to point to the face that "shows how much you hurt". Each facial symbol can be assigned a numerical score (0, 2, 4, 6, 8 and 10) for ease of comparison throughout the hospital course.

What are the considerations for management of supracondylar fractures?

Supracondylar fracture is the most common elbow fracture in children, occurring most commonly in children aged 5–7 years. The fracture is usually caused by a fall on the outstretched hand with the elbow in full extension. Nerve injuries can occur in over 10% of children with this injury, and may be subtle, especially with children <3 years of age, with the median, anterior interosseous, radial and ulnar nerves all potentially involved. Thorough neurological exam, if possible, should be performed at regular time intervals. Similarly, vascular injury can occur, and repeated evaluation of the pulse and color of the hand is essential. Compartment syndrome, while rare, results in devastating complications, and children with displaced supracondylar fractures should be observed for 12–24 h postoperatively to monitor for this complication.

Is regional anesthesia contraindicated in supracondylar fractures?

Regional anesthesia in patients at risk for compartment syndrome is a controversial topic (see Chapter 6). Some argue that subjective symptoms such as pain (the cornerstone of clinical diagnosis for this potentially devastating process) should not be treated with regional techniques for fear of masking worsening ischemia. On the other hand, pain has numerous adverse effects, and, especially in children, can lead to a tremendous amount of long-term psychologic stress and disability if under-treated. There is an absence of data pointing to a causative role of regional anesthesia in compartment syndrome, and, in fact, there are several cases where the diagnosis has been facilitated by regional analgesia, when breakthrough pain alerted the clinician to a change in the patient's condition. Especially in younger children who cannot effectively communicate pain to caregivers, objective monitors such as compartmental pressure monitoring may be a prudent strategy.

Several hours later, the patient is brought to the operating room for closed reduction and internal fixation of the displaced fracture. You decide to perform a regional technique.

Should the block be put in awake or asleep?

Because of the inability of most young children to remain still and/or communicate subjective symptoms such as pain or paresthesia, there is little advantage to performing regional anesthetic techniques in the awake state. Most pediatric anesthesiologists take the stance that the safety benefit of a quiet, immobile child outweighs the potential risk of nerve injury that may or may not be heralded by pain/paresthesia. Several large prospective case series have demonstrated a very low incidence of regional anesthetic complications when performed under general anesthesia. To minimize the risk as much as possible, monitors to decrease the likelihood of intraneural injection should be employed when available, including nerve stimulation, ultrasonography and injection pressure monitoring (discussed in detail in Chapter 17).

Which peripheral nerve blocks are appropriate for elbow surgery?

Traditionally, the interscalene approach to the brachial plexus was felt to be inadequate for elbow (and medial hand) surgery because of sparing of the C8 and T1 nerve roots. However, this can be overcome by performing a "low" interscalene block (one or two fingerbreadths above the clavicle) or by using ultrasound. The ultrasound image will show all of the trunks/roots, and the entire plexus can be anesthetized, if desired, rather than just the superior trunk, as was typically the case for the landmark technique.

The remainder of the brachial plexus approaches (supraclavicular, infraclavicular and axillary) all provide complete coverage for elbow surgery.

You choose to perform an ultrasound-guided supraclavicular block following induction of general anesthesia. What are the technical considerations for this block?

The basic technique for ultrasound-guided supraclavicular block in children is similar to adults. A 38–40-mm linear transducer is an appropriate size for most children, although in very small children and infants, a 25-mm "hockey-stick" compact linear transducer may result in a better "fit" in the supraclavicular fossa.

After sterile skin preparation, the transducer is placed on the supraclavicular fossa at the midpoint of the clavicle, with the probe surface parallel to the plane of the skin (Figure 10.2). The transducer may then be tracked laterally or medially until a bounding subclavian artery is visualized (Figure 10.3). The color Doppler function may aid in locating this landmark (Figure 10.4). The pleura and first rib should be observed as bright white discontinuous lines parallel to the skin surface. These may be differentiated by noting a shadow (rib) or homogeneous lung tissue (pleura) immediately deep to the bright interface. The brachial plexus is located lateral to, and often somewhat superficial to, the subclavian artery, and can be recognized by its hypoechoic "cluster of grapes" appearance.

The recommended approach is in-plane from lateral to medial. An out-of-plane approach directs the needle path at right angles to the pleura, and in small children this can result in pleural puncture quite easily. Needle length is a matter of clinician preference – owing to the shallow depth of the brachial plexus in the supraclavicular fossa, it is sometimes advantageous to make a skin puncture well lateral to the transducer to travel in a shallow, subcutaneous path. A 50-mm needle is acceptable in all but very small children.

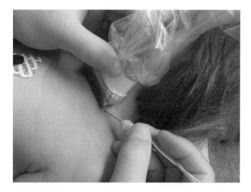

Figure 10.2 Transducer and needle position for ultrasound-guided supraclavicular brachial plexus block in a child.

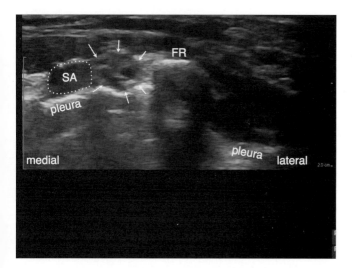

Figure 10.3 Sonoanatomy relevant to the supraclavicular brachial plexus block in a 6-year-old child. Note the pleura and first rib (FR) close to the target brachial plexus (arrows). The subclavian artery (SA) is outlined.

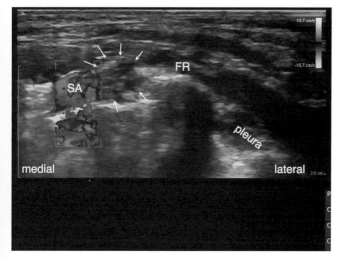

Figure 10.4 The supraclavicular brachial plexus (arrows) in a 6-year-old child with the subclavian artery highlighted using the color Doppler function. FR, First rib; SA, subclavian artery.

Table 10.2 Pediatric dosages for common peripheral nerve blocks

Technique	Dose	Maximum dose
Brachial plexus block	0.3–0.5 ml/kg	15 ml
Rectus sheath block	0.2 ml/kg (per side)	10 ml per side
Ilioinguinal nerve block	0.2 ml/kg	10 ml
Femoral nerve block	0.5 ml/kg	15 ml
Sciatic nerve block	0.5 ml/kg	20 ml

Once the needle tip is adjacent to the brachial plexus, the syringe should be aspirated, and 0.5 ml/kg of a dilute long-acting local anesthetic (e.g. 0.2% ropivacaine) administered slowly with intermittent aspiration, up to a maximum of 15 ml. Since this is an analgesic (not anesthetic) block, it is not critical to place the local anesthetic within the brachial plexus sheath. It is more prudent to err on the side of safety and simply place the local anesthetic next to the plexus.

How should dosing of regional anesthetic blocks be performed in children?

Because children vary in mass substantially, dosages are chosen based on a *milliliter* per kilogram (ml/kg) scheme, with the exception of some small nerves that only require 1–2 ml (e.g. superficial cervical plexus, lateral femoral cutaneous nerve). Examples are outlined in Table 10.2.

The vast majority of blocks in children are analgesic blocks, and do not require the intense motor and sensory blockade required for surgical anesthesia. Ropivacaine 0.2%, levobupivacaine 0.125% or bupivacaine 0.125% are all appropriate choices.

Neonates and young infants (<3–6 months) have reduced levels of plasma cholinesterase, leading to theoretically decreased clearance of ester local anesthetics. This age group also has reduced hepatic bloodflow and immature metabolic degradation pathways, as well as decreased levels of α-1-acid glycoprotein, all of which increase plasma levels of amide local anesthetics and put the infant at higher risk for systemic toxicity. For this reason, the following infusion rates are recommended (note that units are in *milligrams* per kilogram per hour):

- For neonates and infants: 0.2 mg/kg/h of ropivacaine 0.1%

- For older children: 0.3–0.4 mg/kg/h of ropivacaine 0.1%.

Further reading

Abzug, J. M., Herman, M. J. (2012). Management of supracondylar humerus fractures in children: current concepts. *The Journal of the American Academy of Orthopaedic Surgeons*, **20**, 69–77.

Amiri, H. R., Espandar, R. (2011). Upper extremity surgery in younger children under ultrasound-guided supraclavicular brachial plexus block: a case series. *Journal of Children's Orthopaedics*, **5**, 5–9.

De José María, B., Banús, E., Navarro Egea, M. et al. (2008). Ultrasound-guided supraclavicular vs infraclavicular brachial plexus blocks in children. *Paediatric Anaesthesia*, **18**, 838–44.

Drendel, A. L., Kelly, B. T., Ali, S. (2011). Pain assessment for children: overcoming challenges and optimizing care. *Pediatric Emergency Care*, **27**, 773–81.

Gadsden, J. C., Tsai, T., Iwata, T. et al. (2009). Low interscalene block provides reliable anesthesia for surgery at or about the elbow. *Journal of Clinical Anesthesia*, **21**, 98–102.

Petrowsky, H., Raeder, S., Zuercher, L. et al. (2012). A quarter century experience in liver trauma: a plea for early computed tomography and conservative management for all hemodynamically stable patients. *World Journal of Surgery*, **36**, 247–54.

Wolf, A. R. (2012). Effects of regional analgesia on stress responses to pediatric surgery. *Paediatric Anaesthesia*, **22**, 19–24.

Yang, C. W., Cho, C.-K., Kwon, H. U. et al. (2010). Ultrasound-guided supraclavicular brachial plexus block in pediatric patients – a report of four cases. *Korean Journal of Anesthesiology*, **59** Suppl, S90–4.

Regional anesthesia for fractured neck of femur

Key aspects of case

1. The effect of regional analgesia on postoperative delirium.
2. Evidence base for morbidity and mortality outcomes in hip fracture patients using regional anesthetic techniques.

Case presentation

An 81-year-old woman presents to the emergency room with right hip pain after tripping over her cat while walking to the kitchen. She did not lose consciousness and has no other injuries of note due to the fall. She lives alone but has a home aide visit her three times/week for help with housekeeping and shopping. Her daughter states that she is "mostly there" mentally, but has become a little forgetful in recent years. Her past medical history includes hypertension and atrial fibrillation, for which she takes metoprolol, diltiazem and warfarin. On examination, her right leg is shortened and externally rotated, and she is loudly complaining of severe pain. Her lab work reveals a hemoglobin of 12 g/dl, and an international normalized ratio (INR) of 1.5.

Case discussion

How is acute pain commonly treated for hip fracture in the emergency department?

Neck of femur (NOF) fractures are more common in the elderly and in females, and are associated with long-term functional impairment and a reduced quality of life. Despite the fact that many of these patients present in moderate to severe pain, a significant number of patients with hip fracture receive little or no analgesic intervention prehospital or in the emergency department, and those that do may wait hours for relief. Factors contributing to "oligoanalgesia" include patient confusion, concern regarding side effects in a cohort with multiple comorbidities, inadequate pain assessment and language/communication breakdown.

Opioids remain the mainstay (>50%) of analgesic therapy for hip fracture despite the long list of side effects, such as respiratory depression, constipation, urinary retention, and nausea and vomiting. Other systemic drugs, such as acetaminophen, NSAIDs and codeine, are less common, as are nerve blocks, with a documented nerve block rate of 7% in one survey of 36 Australian hospitals.

Does the use of regional analgesia for relieving acute pain associated with hip fracture impact the risk of developing delirium?

Delirium is a common finding in the elderly hospitalized patient, especially in the post-operative setting, and is an independent risk factor for death, institutionalization and dementia. Opioids are well known to contribute to delirium in the elderly and their use should be minimized if possible. On the other hand, moderate to severe pain is also a risk factor for delirium. The role that regional analgesic techniques play in reducing the incidence of cognitive dysfunction has historically been somewhat unclear, relating to the complex pathophysiology. Several studies and reviews have compared neuraxial versus general anesthesia with respect to cognitive outcome and found no difference in incidence. One key methodologic flaw to many of these studies, however, is the absence of preoperative or postoperative regional analgesic intervention. It is not difficult to understand why 1 hour of spinal anesthesia might not make a difference for acute fracture pain that lasts for days to weeks.

Prolonged nerve blockade may be more effective than a single intervention. Mouzopoulos et al. (2009) found that hip fracture patients at moderate risk for delirium who received daily fascia iliaca blocks before and after operation had a significantly reduced incidence of delirium than those who were randomized to placebo. Similarly, elective hip replacement patients randomized to continuous lumbar plexus or femoral catheters had significantly reduced serious delirium or confusion compared to systemic analgesia post-operatively in a study by Marino et al. (2009) (0%, 1.3% and 10.7%, respectively). Outcomes such as these support the idea that regional analgesia should be initiated as soon as possible for these high-risk patients and continued until the intensity of pain is low enough to justify halting the block.

Describe the technical aspects of placing an ultrasound-guided femoral block

Typically this block is performed in the supine position, with the bed or table flattened to maximize access to the inguinal area. The skin is disinfected and the transducer positioned over the midpoint of the inguinal crease (Figure 11.1). The transducer can then be moved laterally or medially to find the femoral artery and vein, which are obvious landmarks. The color Doppler function may help in locating these landmarks.

The nerve should appear as a bright, flattened triangle or oval just lateral and deep to the femoral artery (Figure 11.2). If not immediately apparent, toggling or tilting the trans-ducer proximally or distally can often help to improve the contrast and bring the nerve "out" of the background. The nerve is wedged in between the iliacus muscle and the femoral artery, and is often best seen at the level of the artery's bifurcation. This can be elicited by moving the transducer caudad and cephalad along its course.

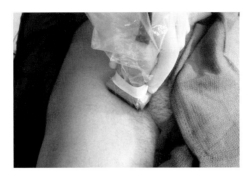

Figure 11.1 Transducer position for ultrasound-guided femoral nerve block.

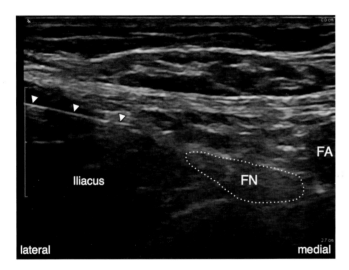

Figure 11.2 Sonoanatomy relevant to femoral nerve block. Note the femoral nerve (FN) sandwiched between the iliacus muscle and the femoral artery (FA). The needle (arrowheads) is approaching from the lateral side.

Once identified, a skin wheal is made on the lateral aspect of the thigh 1 cm away from the lateral edge of the transducer. The needle is then inserted in-plane in a lateral-to-medial orientation and advanced towards the femoral nerve. If nerve stimulation is used, the passage of the needle through the fascia iliaca and contact of the needle tip with the femoral nerve is usually associated with a motor response of the quadriceps muscle group.

Once the needle tip is visualized adjacent to the nerve, the syringe is aspirated and 1–2 ml of local anesthetic is injected to confirm proper location. Femoral nerve block requires 15–20 ml of local anesthetic in adults, but less volume may be sufficient for proper spread (Figure 11.3). While a single injection of such volumes of local anesthetic suffices, it may be beneficial to inject two or three smaller doses at different locations (i.e. posterior and lateral) to improve the speed of onset of the block.

The patient is scheduled by the orthopedic surgery service for urgent percutaneous hip pinning in the supine position. They estimate a surgical time of 40 minutes.

Table 11.1 Summary of randomized controlled trials comparing neuraxial versus general anesthesia for hip fracture surgery since 1990

Study	n	Groups	Regional outcome
Adams et al. (1990)	56	Spinal GA with ETT	Spinal attenuated ↑ in norepinephrine, ADH No difference in mortality, other outcomes
Biffoli et al. (1998)	60	Spinal GA with ETT	No difference in postoperative mental status
Casati et al. (2003)	30	Spinal GA with LMA	Faster discharge from PACU No difference in hypotension, cognition
Juelsgaard et al. (1998)	43	Titrated continuous spinal Single-dose spinal GA with ETT	Hypotension and myocardial ischemia reduced in continuous spinal group No difference in mortality

GA, General anesthesia; ETT, endotracheal tube; ADH, antidiuretic hormone; LMA, laryngeal mask airway; PACU, post-anesthesia care unit.

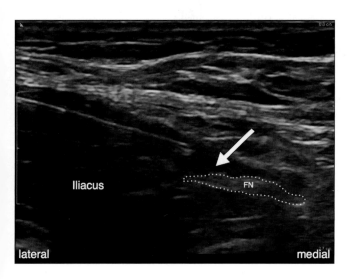

Figure 11.3 Femoral nerve (FN) and surrounding structures following injection of local anesthetic. Note that, in comparison to Figure 11.2, the nerve has peeled away from the overlying fascia iliaca, and a pool of local anesthetic now lies between these two structures.

Does the choice of neuraxial over general anesthesia result in improved outcomes?

The influence of general versus neuraxial anesthesia on outcomes for hip fracture surgery is controversial. The principal problems in the existing literature are heterogeneity in study design, patient population and procedure type, which precludes a meaningful overall conclusion. There are only a handful of recent (since 1990) randomized controlled studies that examine the effect of anesthetic technique on outcome for hip fracture surgery specifically (Table 11.1). While post-anesthesia care unit (PACU) discharge time, hypotension and myocardial ischemia appear to be reduced with neuraxial techniques, these results must be interpreted with caution, as they are small, single studies.

On the other hand, a slightly less strict evaluation (i.e. including studies of elective hip surgery and those with non-randomized designs) leads to similarly encouraging results. For example, larger meta-analyses and systematic reviews (e.g. Urwin et al., 2000; Parker et al., 2004d; Luger et al., 2010) have shown reductions in the incidence of deep venous thrombosis and postoperative confusion, as well as a tendency to fewer myocardial infarctions, less pneumonia, fewer fatal pulmonary embolisms and less postoperative hypoxia. Neuman et al. (2012) found that regional anesthesia was associated with a 25–29% reduction in pulmonary complications and death in one review of more than 18 000 hip fracture patients. Luger et al. (2010) stated that regional anesthesia "is the technique of choice (although) the limited evidence available do(es) not permit a definitive conclusion to be drawn with regard to mortality or other outcomes." Recently, the Association of Anaesthetists of Great Britain and Ireland published a guideline for the management of patients with hip fractures. The Working Party's position was that, until such time as evidence is published that confirms that regional anesthesia is superior to general anesthesia or vice versa, neuraxial anesthesia should be considered for all patients undergoing hip fracture repair, unless contraindicated. Ultimately, careful attention to the patient's comorbidities and physiologic reserve is likely a more important determinant of postoperative outcome than anesthetic technique.

Can hip surgery be performed under peripheral nerve block alone?

While neuraxial anesthesia remains the most popular method for open reduction and internal fixation (ORIF) of hip fractures, peripheral nerve block (PNB) techniques have been described. The hip is supplied primarily by the branches of the lumbar plexus (femoral and obturator nerves), as is the skin overlying the trochanter (lateral femoral cutaneous nerve). Some clinicians state that lumbar plexus block provides "enough" anesthesia, as some local anesthetic may distribute in a caudal direction to block the lumbosacral trunk. However, articular branches also arise from the sacral plexus, namely the superior gluteal nerve, the nerve to quadratus femoris as well as directly from the sciatic nerve. As a result, a proximal sciatic nerve block should be performed to ensure complete anesthesia. The more proximal the approach, the more likely the sacral plexus will be blocked – for example, a parasacral approach almost always anesthetizes the sacral plexus, whereas the posterior (Labat) approach may miss some of the articular twigs from the smaller nerves.

Since these nerve blocks are not beginner-level blocks, and the lumbar plexus block in particular is not without risk, there should be a good reason to choose this technique over a spinal (e.g. aortic stenosis). A good compromise that achieves most of the goals for this case might be a spinal anesthetic followed by the placement of a lumbar plexus catheter for postoperative pain, both performed in the lateral position.

Does the patient's elevated INR preclude the use of neuraxial anesthesia/analgesia?

The risk of spinal hematoma following neuraxial blockade in patients who are coagulopathic is largely unknown, and recommendations regarding thresholds for avoiding spinal or epidural techniques are based on consensus opinion. In general, a factor VII activity level of 40% is associated with adequate hemostasis. Since factor VII is the vitamin-K-dependent clotting factor with the shortest half-life and an INR of 1.5 reflects an activity level of >40%, many believe that it is safe to administer neuraxial anesthesia if the INR is <1.5 (e.g. The American Society of Regional Anesthesia and Pain Medicine Consensus Conference Guidelines). The European Society of Regional Anesthesia advocates an acceptable threshold of <1.4.

However, there are clearly substantial benefits to neuraxial anesthesia and analgesia, and these must be weighed carefully against the potential risks. For example, the Scandinavian Society of Anaesthesiology and Intensive Care Medicine has issued a thoughtful document on this issue (Breivik *et al.*, 2010) that stratifies the recommended INR threshold based on the expected benefit: if a spinal is being considered for comfort only, the recommended maximum INR should be ≤1.4. However, if it is being used in a situation where it has been shown to decrease morbidity, that threshold increases to <1.8; if expected to reduce mortality, it increases again to <2.2. Because the incidence of spinal hematoma is larger with epidural and combined spinal–epidural, these respective thresholds are ≤1.2, <1.6 and <1.8.

References and further reading

Adams, H. A., Wolf, C., Michaelis, G., Hempelmann, G. (1990). [Postoperative course and endocrine stress reaction of geriatric patients with para-articular hip fractures. Prospective randomized study comparing spinal anesthesia and halothane intubation narcosis]. *Anästhesie, Intensivtherapie, Notfallmedizin*, **25**, 263–70.

Beaudoin, F. L., Nagdev, A., Merchant, R. C., Becker, B. M. (2010). Ultrasound-guided femoral nerve blocks in elderly patients with hip fractures. *The American Journal of Emergency Medicine*, **28**, 76–81.

Biffoli, F., Piacentino, V., Meconcelli, G et al. (1998). [The effect of anesthesiologic technique on the mental state of elderly patients submitted for orthopedic surgery of the lower limbs]. *Minerva Anestesiologica*, **64**, 13–19.

Breivik, H., Bang, U., Jalonen, J. et al. (2010). Nordic guidelines for neuraxial blocks in disturbed haemostasis from the Scandinavian Society of Anaesthesiology and Intensive Care Medicine. *Acta Anaesthesiologica Scandinavica*, **54**, 16–41.

Casati, A., Aldegheri, G., Vinciguerra, E. et al. (2003). Randomized comparison between sevoflurane anaesthesia and unilateral spinal anaesthesia in elderly patients undergoing orthopaedic surgery. *European Journal of Anaesthesiology*, **20**, 640–6.

Gadsden J, Todd K. Regional anesthesia and acute pain management in the emergency department. In: Hadzic, A. (2006). *Textbook of Regional Anesthesia and Acute Pain Management*, 1st edn. New York: McGraw-Hill Professional, pp. 955–66.

Griffiths, R., Alper, J., Beckingsale, A. et al. (2012). Management of proximal femoral fractures 2011: Association of Anaesthetists of Great Britain and Ireland. *Anaesthesia*, **67**, 85–98.

Ho, A. M. H., Karmakar, M. K. (2002). Combined paravertebral lumbar plexus and parasacral sciatic nerve block for reduction of hip fracture in a patient with severe aortic stenosis. *Canadian Journal of Anaesthesia*, **49**, 946–50.

Holdgate, A., Shepherd, S. A., Huckson, S. (2010). Patterns of analgesia for fractured neck of femur in Australian emergency departments. *Emergency Medicine Australasia: EMA*, **22**, 3–8.

Juelsgaard, P., Sand, N. P., Felsby, S. et al. (1998). Perioperative myocardial ischaemia in patients undergoing surgery for fractured hip randomized to incremental spinal, single-dose spinal or general anaesthesia. *European Journal of Anaesthesiology*, **15**, 656–63.

Luger, T. J., Kammerlander, C., Gosch, M. *et al.* (2010). Neuroaxial versus general anaesthesia in geriatric patients for hip fracture surgery: does it matter? *Osteoporosis International*, **21**, S555–72.

Marino, J., Russo, J., Kenny, M. *et al.* (2009). Continuous lumbar plexus block for postoperative pain control after total hip arthroplasty. A randomized controlled trial. *The Journal of Bone and Joint Surgery. American Volume*, **91**, 29–37.

Mouzopoulos, G., Vasiliadis, G., Lasanianos, N. *et al.* (2009). Fascia iliaca block prophylaxis for hip fracture patients at risk for delirium: a randomized placebo-controlled study.

Journal of Orthopaedics and Traumatology, **10**, 127–33.

Neuman, M. D., Silber, J. H., Elkassabany, N. M. *et al.* (2012). Comparative effectiveness of regional versus general anesthesia for hip fracture surgery in adults. *Anesthesiology*, **117**, 72–92.

Parker, M. J., Handoll, H. H. G., Griffiths, R. (2004). Anaesthesia for hip fracture surgery in adults. *Cochrane Database of Systematic Reviews (Online)*, (**4**), CD000521.

Urwin, S. C., Parker, M. J., Griffiths, R. (2000). General versus regional anaesthesia for hip fracture surgery: a meta-analysis of randomized trials. *British Journal of Anaesthesia*, **84**, 450–5.

Regional anesthesia in the intoxicated trauma patient

Key aspects of case

1. Consent for regional anesthetic techniques in trauma.
2. Peripheral nerve blocks of the arm and forearm.

Case presentation

A 23-year-old male walks into the emergency department after being involved in a brawl at a local bar. He is clearly intoxicated and is arguing with the paramedics and nursing staff. His injuries include an open displaced fracture of his right fifth metacarpal and a disloca-tion of the left first carpometacarpal (CMC) joint, along with various superficial cuts and bruises. He is maintaining his own airway, is hemodynamically stable and has no other injuries. He is otherwise healthy and has been eating bar food as recently as 1 hour ago. Because of the open nature of the fifth metacarpal fracture, he is booked for urgent debride-ment and percutaneous fixation of the fracture, as well as closed reduction of the CMC dislocation.

Case discussion

What are the anesthetic options for this case?

Factors that will determine the appropriate choice of anesthetic technique in trauma include concomitant injuries, airway concerns (including stability of the cervical spine), the ability to lie still during a regional technique, evidence of neurologic impairment and the presence of other contraindications to neural blockade such as profound hypovolemia, coagulopathy, etc.

In this patient, general anesthesia is preferred because of his combative behavior and the need to operate on two distant sites. Moreover, his airway and cervical spine are not injured and can be managed with little additional difficulty (apart from his full stomach status). Peripheral nerve blocks (PNBs) may be placed before or after the induction of general anesthesia (see Chapter 17) for postoperative pain control. The pain intensity associated with a fifth metacarpal fracture is probably not severe enough to warrant a long-duration catheter technique, and a single-injection block is usually sufficient. Bilateral intravenous regional anesthesia is a poor choice owing to the risk of systemic toxicity.

What are the issues surrounding consent in the trauma patient for regional anesthetic/analgesic procedures?

Informed consent is a process that consists of three elements: (1) an explanation of the procedure/therapy as well as the alternatives, and the risks and benefits of both; (2) patient comprehension of the proposed procedure/therapy; and (3) mutual agreement between doctor and patient. While this is an acceptable paradigm for elective procedures, the process of informed consent is often different in the traumatically injured population. First and foremost, these patients are frequently in moderate to severe pain, are psychologically distressed, have received sedative medications, and can be neurologically impaired, either from the injury itself or from drugs and/or alcohol. This presents a substantial challenge to the requirement that a patient has the capacity to make an informed decision. However, mild sedation and opioid analgesia has been shown not to impair the patient's ability to recall important elements of the informed consent after the procedure.

Clearly, if the patient's condition is so critical that emergency surgery is warranted, or if no proxy decision-maker is present, consent can be waived, as it is implied that the patient would desire a life- or limb-saving procedure unless stated explicitly otherwise. This intoxicated patient obviously cannot fully appreciate the risks and benefits of the proposed procedure, and is unable to consent; on the other hand, his open fracture presents a risk for complications, and should be irrigated and repaired within 6–8 hours. This is a controversial area, and, while some physicians would obtain informed consent from a proxy decision-maker and proceed with the operation, some would elect to defer until the next day until the patient was fully capable, depending on his/her assessment of the relative risk of delay.

In contrast to general anesthesia, regional anesthetic or analgesic interventions are rarely "required" to facilitate life- or limb-saving procedures. Despite their myriad advantages for postoperative pain control and effects on morbidity and mortality in some cases, there are few indications for an "emergency" nerve block. As such, the threshold for acceptable consent conditions must be high – many anesthesiologists would not accept the admittedly rare risk of causing a nerve injury in this patient before having the opportunity to explain the procedure fully. This is especially true for injuries and procedures that are associated with mild to moderate pain that can be treated with acetaminophen, NSAIDs and mild opioid analgesic medications. An acceptable strategy if a nerve block is still desired might be to temporize with systemic medications until the patient is no longer intoxicated, at which time the possibility of blocks can be raised.

On the other hand, the risk of permanent nerve injury or other complication from a PNB in this situation is very rare, and allows the physician to provide excellent analgesia, reduce opioid usage and proceed with a "light" general anesthetic in an effort to reduce side effects. The avoidance of additional drugs that obscure mentation is particularly important in cases where frequent neurologic status assessments are required, such as closed head injury.

What are the advantages and disadvantages of various peripheral nerve block approaches for hand surgery?

Approaches anywhere along the brachial plexus from the roots/trunks through to the terminal branches can be utilized effectively for hand surgery. Because the operative area is small and is innervated by a limited number of nerves, and because profound motor and sensory block

Table 12.1 Regional anesthetic options for hand surgery

Block approach	Advantages	Disadvantages
Interscalene brachial plexus	Complete hand anesthesia (providing all trunks are blocked; occasionally miss inferior trunk, especially with nerve stimulator technique) Easy, shallow technique	May miss ulnar nerve (especially with nerve stimulator technique) Unnecessary upper arm sensory/motor block Side effects: phrenic nerve palsy, Horner's syndrome, recurrent laryngeal nerve palsy
Supraclavicular brachial plexus	Complete hand anesthesia Easy, shallow technique	Unnecessary upper arm sensory/motor block Side effects: possible phrenic nerve palsy, unknown incidence of pneumothorax
Infraclavicular brachial plexus	Complete hand anesthesia	Unnecessary upper arm sensory/motor block Deeper block, somewhat more challenging Potential for pneumothorax Caution with anticoagulation
Axillary brachial plexus	Complete hand anesthesia Easy, shallow technique Can select individual nerves No risk of pneumothorax	Unnecessary upper arm sensory/motor block Increased risk of vascular puncture, hematoma If musculocutaneous nerve block is required, may require separate block, although not challenging
Distal terminal branches	Very easy, especially with ultrasound Only anesthetize the areas required; no unnecessary arm sensory/motor block Very small volumes of local anesthetic required → reduced systemic toxicity risk	May require supplementation with field blocks if incision extends proximal to wrist crease

of the shoulder and upper arm are not required, a more distal approach is often preferred at our institution (Table 12.1). This allows the patient to be discharged immediately without a sling because the biceps brachii muscle is not affected.

What is the best location to perform ultrasound-guided terminal branch blocks in the upper limb?

Because of their relatively shallow course in the distal arm and forearm, the median, ulnar and radial nerves are easily blocked in multiple locations at or distal to the elbow. One limiting factor can be dressings or casts, but in most cases these can be removed at the time of surgery to expose the block site.

Sonographically, the best place to visualize each nerve is at a level where it cannot be confused with tendons, ligaments or other fascial tissues, as they can look very similar. This tends to make ultrasound-guided blocks at the elbow and wrist creases an unpopular

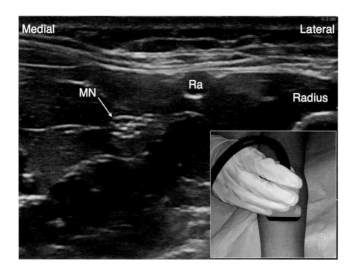

Figure 12.1 The transducer position and sonoanatomy for ultrasound-guided median nerve block in the forearm. MN, Median nerve; Ra, radial artery.

choice. Instead, the easiest location to visualize these nerves is at a location where nothing but muscle surrounds them.

The median nerve can be easily visualized in the mid-forearm with the ultrasound transducer placed on the volar aspect (Figure 12.1). The nerve can be seen as a bright oval with dark interior stippling (fascicles) in the center of the forearm, deep to the flexor digitorum superficialis muscle. Frequently, some tilting of the transducer is required to "bring out" the nerve from the background. To confirm that the structure is a nerve and not an intramuscular tendon, it should be traced several centimeters distally and proximally.

The ulnar nerve is also best visualized in the mid-forearm, on the ulnar (medial) aspect of the ulnar artery, taking on a similar appearance to the median nerve (Figure 12.2.). Tracing the artery and nerve proximally several centimeters should result in the artery separating and traveling deeper, while the nerve remains in a shallow position. This may represent a safer place to block the nerve, as the likelihood of arterial puncture is reduced.

The radial nerve is best imaged just proximal to the lateral epicondyle in between the brachialis (deep) and brachioradialis (superficial) muscles (Figure 12.3). While some clinicians advocate blocking the superficial branch of the nerve in the forearm, its course is usually intimately associated with the radial artery, and, to avoid the risk of arterial puncture altogether, this more proximal approach is used in our practice.

For each of these nerves, their ease of identification, lack of vulnerable structures nearby and shallow depth allow the clinician the choice of any needle approach. In-plane and out-of-plane are both effective. Each nerve only requires 3–5 ml of local anesthetic to obtain an excellent block. The choice of local anesthetic depends on the procedure. For surgical anesthesia in a quick hand procedure with minimal expected postoperative pain, lidocaine or mepivacaine (1.5–2%) might be best. Ropivacaine, bupivacaine or levo-bupivacaine 0.2–0.5% can be used if a prolonged duration is warranted.

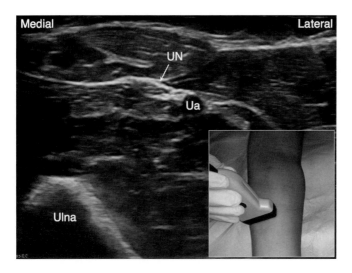

Figure 12.2 The transducer position and sonoanatomy for ultrasound-guided ulnar nerve block in the forearm. Ua, Ulnar artery; UN, ulnar nerve.

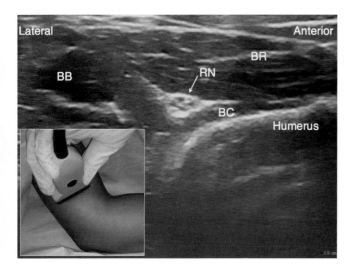

Figure 12.3 The transducer position and sonoanatomy for ultrasound-guided radial nerve block in the distal arm. BB, Biceps brachii muscle; BC, brachialis muscle; BR, brachioradialis muscle; RN, radial nerve.

What nerves need to be anesthetized to perform fifth finger pinning?

The fifth finger is innervated by fibers originating from the eighth cervical root (C8) that contribute, along with fibers from T1, to the formation of the ulnar nerve. For this reason, and because there is no contribution from the radial or median nerves, any procedure on the fifth finger can be performed with a simple ulnar nerve block (Figure 12.4). Note that if the incision extends more proximally than the wrist crease on the ulnar side, a blockade of

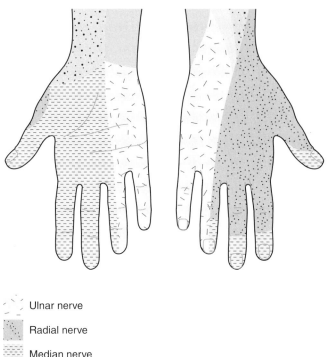

Figure 12.4 Dermatomes of the volar and dorsal surfaces of the hand.

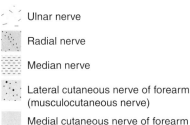

Ulnar nerve

Radial nerve

Median nerve

Lateral cutaneous nerve of forearm (musculocutaneous nerve)

Medial cutaneous nerve of forearm

the medial cutaneous nerve of the forearm should be performed, which is easily done as a simple subcutaneous field block just distal to the elbow crease.

How much local anesthetic is required to anesthetize each nerve?

Some investigators have found that volumes as low as <1 ml are sufficient to block a terminal nerve in the forearm. However, for practical purposes, we routinely use at least 3–5 ml per nerve to ensure a semicircular spread around the nerve (Figure 12.5). This also ensures that block setup is rapid, with minimal delay in ability of the surgeon to start the case.

The surgeon attempts to reduce the left first CMC dislocation but it remains unstable. She states that she would like to place a pin through the joint to stabilize it.

Which peripheral nerves need to be blocked for this procedure? What about other digits?

The thumb is innervated by both the median and radial nerves, and both need to be blocked to provide surgical anesthesia for this procedure. Similarly, procedures on the second finger would require both median and radial nerve blockade.

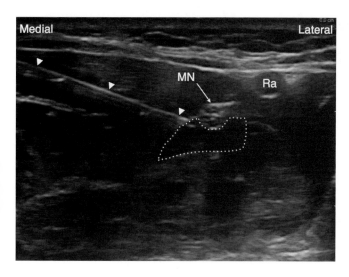

Figure 12.5 Ultrasound-guided median nerve block. The needle (arrowheads) has been advanced in-plane until the tip is adjacent to the nerve (MN) and 5 ml of local anesthetic deposited, which can be seen deep to the nerve (outlined portion). Ra, Radial artery.

The third and fourth fingers are variably innervated by all three nerves. Despite classic textbook images of the fourth finger being "split" down the volar surface by the median and ulnar nerves, there is considerable variation in the innervation to either digit, and, to ensure complete anesthesia for these digits, blockade of the median, ulnar and radial nerves is recommended. Because the volume of local anesthetic used for each individual nerve is so low, the risk of systemic toxicity is minimal and the downside to "hedging your bets" by blocking all the nerves is negligible.

Further reading

Brull, R., McCartney, C. J. L., Chan, V. W. S. *et al.* (2007). Disclosure of risks associated with regional anesthesia: a survey of academic regional anesthesiologists. *Regional Anesthesia and Pain Medicine*, **32**, 7–11.

Eichenberger, U., Stöckli, S., Marhofer, P. *et al.* (2009). Minimal local anesthetic volume for peripheral nerve block: a new ultrasound-guided, nerve dimension-based method. *Regional Anesthesia and Pain Medicine*, **34**, 242–6.

Gianesello, L., Pavoni, V., Coppini, R. *et al.* (2010). Comfort and satisfaction during axillary brachial plexus block in trauma patients: comparison of techniques. *Journal of Clinical Anesthesia*, **22**, 7–12.

Green, D. S. T., MacKenzie, C. R. (2007). Nuances of informed consent: the paradigm of regional anesthesia. *HSS Journal: The Musculoskeletal Journal of Hospital for Special Surgery*, **3**, 115–18.

Liebmann, O., Price, D., Mills, C. *et al.* (2006). Feasibility of forearm ultrasonography-guided nerve blocks of the radial, ulnar, and median nerves for hand procedures in the emergency department. *Annals of Emergency Medicine*, **48**, 558–62.

McCartney, C. J. L., Xu, D., Constantinescu, C., Abbas, S., Chan, V. W. S. (2007). Ultrasound examination of peripheral nerves in the forearm. *Regional Anesthesia and Pain Medicine*, **32**, 434–9.

Smith, H. K., Manjaly, J. G., Yousri, T. *et al.* (2011). Informed consent in trauma: Does written information improve patient recall of risks? A prospective randomised study. *Injury*. doi:10.1016/j.injury.2011.06.419

Regional anesthesia for humeral shaft fracture

Key aspects of case

1. Considerations for regional anesthesia in the patient at risk for neurologic deficits.
2. Interscalene brachial plexus catheters.

Case presentation

A 35-year-old, right-handed factory worker is loading materials onto a shelf when the shelving unit tips over, pinning his left arm underneath it. He is extricated immediately and brought by ambulance to hospital where he is diagnosed with an open midshaft humeral fracture. He is awake and breathing spontaneously, with no tenderness of his cervical spine and full range of motion. He has no other injuries and is hemodynamically stable. On questioning, he states that he has 7/10 pain in his arm, but examination of the left forearm and hand reveal no gross neurologic deficits or vascular compromise.

Case discussion

What are the considerations in the management of humeral shaft fractures?

Humeral fractures comprise 3% of all fractures and most commonly occur in the midshaft. If closed and not severely displaced, these are usually treated with functional bracing, which has a very good outcome with minimal disability or deformity. Indications for surgical treatment include open fractures, vascular injury, intra-articular fractures and ipsilateral ulnar fracture. This is usually accomplished by application of a plate, although intramedullary nailing is also performed, often for pathologic or segmental fractures.

Radial nerve palsy is present in 16% of humeral shaft fractures. The presentation is typically wrist drop, weakness of finger extension and paresthesias along the dorsum of the forearm and hand. Elbow extension is preserved generally, as the motor branches to the triceps muscle originate prior to the spiral groove. Radial nerve palsy by itself is not an indication for operative treatment, although most orthopedic surgeons will operate when it presents in combination with an open fracture. Recovery is complete in >85% of cases at 6 months.

The orthopedic surgeon has scheduled the patient for an anterior plating of the fracture, and asks that you provide general anesthesia so that he can assess the radial nerve function immediately postoperatively.

What is the anatomic basis for radial nerve injury in humeral shaft fracture?

The radial nerve originates from the posterior cord in the axilla before winding around the humerus at midshaft in the spiral groove between the lateral and medial head of the triceps muscle. Approximately 10 cm from the elbow crease, it pierces the lateral intermuscular septum and runs between the brachioradialis and brachialis muscles, emerging above the lateral epicondyle. It is the intimate association with the humeral shaft in the spiral groove that predisposes the nerve to either compression injuries ("Saturday night palsy") or traction/laceration injuries, as in this case.

Besides the original injury, surgical repair of humeral fractures have also been associated with radial nerve injuries owing to the close association of the nerve to the humerus along the midshaft. Dissection and retraction of the muscles and nerve must be done with care so as not to crush, stretch or otherwise traumatize the nerve.

Postoperatively, the surgeon evaluates the patient and finds him to have intact neurologic function. He is prescribed IV morphine patient-controlled analgesia and discharged to the floor. On postoperative day 1, the patient complains of unrelenting pain despite the morphine, and the surgeon consults you with a view to performing a longlasting regional analgesic technique.

You decide to do an ultrasound-guided interscalene brachial plexus catheter. What are the technical considerations for performing this technique?

The chief advantage of ultrasound guidance for interscalene block is not block success – clinicians relatively skilled at landmark and nerve stimulation techniques already enjoy a near 100% success rate. Rather, it is the ability to visualize and target specific elements of the brachial plexus (e.g. the superior trunk), and therefore: (1) reduce the volume of local anesthetic used; (2) avoid inadvertent side effects usually associated with large-volume interscalene block (e.g. Horner's syndrome, recurrent laryngeal nerve block); and (3) avoid complications such as arterial, pleural or neural puncture.

Typically, the block is performed with the patient in a semilateral position, with the patient's head turned away from the side to be blocked (Figure 13.1). This is ergonomically more convenient, especially during an in-plane approach from the lateral side, in which the

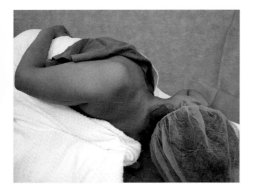

Figure 13.1 Semilateral position prior to performing an ultrasound-guided interscalene brachial plexus block.

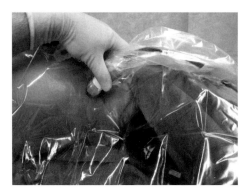

Figure 13.2 Transducer position for ultrasound-guided interscalene brachial plexus block.

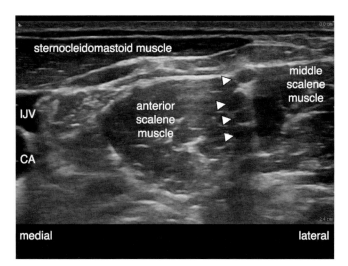

Figure 13.3 Sonoanatomy relevant to ultrasound-guided interscalene brachial plexus block. The roots and/or trunks of the brachial plexus (arrowheads) are sandwiched between the anterior and middle scalene muscles. CA, Carotid artery; IJV, internal jugular vein.

needle is entering the skin at the posterolateral aspect of the neck. A slight elevation of the head of the bed is often more comfortable for the patient.

With the patient in the correct position, the skin is disinfected, sterile drapes applied and the transducer is positioned just above the clavicle at its midpoint in the transverse plane (Figure 13.2). The transducer is then slid laterally or medially to identify the subclavian artery and the brachial plexus just lateral to it. This often appears as a bundle of dark (hypoechoic) ovals. Keeping an eye on the plexus, the transducer is then slowly moved in a cephalad direction about 4–5 cm, or until a characteristic image of the interscalene brachial plexus is achieved. This should include the anterior and middle scalene muscles, and a "string" of 3–5 dark nodules in between (Figure 13.3). Cervical fascia and sternocleidomastoid muscles are seen superficial to the plexus. The brachial plexus is typically visualized at 1–3 cm depth.

A 50-mm insulated 17-GA Tuohy needle is then inserted in-plane towards the brachial plexus, typically in a lateral-to-medial direction (Figure 13.4), although medial-to-lateral needle approach, or an out-of-plane approach can also be chosen if more convenient. As the needle passes through the perimysium of the middle scalene muscle, a palpable "give" is often appreciated, indicating that the needle tip has entered the brachial plexus sheath. Care must

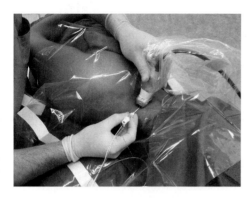

Figure 13.4 Transducer and needle position for ultrasound-guided continuous interscalene brachial plexus block.

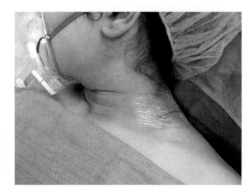

Figure 13.5 Catheter securement technique for ultrasound-guided continuous interscalene brachial plexus block. Note the catheter emerges from the skin and is taped away from the surgical field, around the back of the neck, and adhered to the contralateral chest wall for easy and safe access.

be taken not to advance the needle directly at a nerve trunk, as nerves at the interscalene level are especially susceptible to mechanical injury. Instead, the needle can usually be directed to enter the sheath between the superior and middle trunk. When nerve stimulation is used (0.5 mA, 0.1 ms), the entrance of the needle is often associated with a motor response of the shoulder, arm or forearm.

After careful aspiration, 1–2 ml of local anesthetic is injected to document the proper needle tip location. A further 5–7 ml is used to "open up" the space for the catheter. The transducer can then be put down momentarily while the catheter is advanced 1–2 cm beyond the tip of the needle. Alternatively, if a helper is present, he/she can advance the catheter with sterile gloves while its course is followed on the ultrasound monitor. Once the needle is removed, the final catheter tip position should be evaluated by observing the appropriate spread of additional local anesthetic, or with the use of the color Doppler function.

The skin of the neck is mobile and there is a tendency for catheters to become displaced if not secured adequately. A small amount of topical adhesive such as Dermabond™ will ensure that infusate does not leak out of the puncture site. The catheter should then be taped or secured with Tegaderm™ around the back of the neck to the contralateral side, which keeps it out of the surgical field and permits access for additional boluses during surgery (Figure 13.5).

An infusion of long-acting local anesthetic (e.g. ropivacaine 0.2%, bupivacaine or levo-bupivacaine 0.125%) can be delivered at a rate of 5 ml/h, with a 5-ml patient-controlled bolus every 30–45 minutes.

The patient's pain is well controlled after the catheter is placed. After 48 h the infusion is stopped in preparation for discharge home. The nurse notices that the patient has reduced power in wrist extension compared with the right side. When asked, he states that he also has decreased sensation over the dorsum of his hand, despite return of function of sensation in the median and ulnar territories.

What is "double-crush" syndrome?

The "double-crush" syndrome is a condition that is believed to occur when axons, having been compressed at one point along their course, are especially susceptible to damage at another site. For instance, a patient with thoracic outlet obstruction and a subclinical brachial plexopathy may not report any symptoms or nerve dysfunction; however, if the same patient develops an otherwise undetectable carpal tunnel syndrome, the combined neurologic insult presents clinically. Not all double-crush syndromes are mechanical in nature; other potential insults include metabolic (e.g. diabetes mellitus, HIV), ischemic (e.g. peripheral vascular disease), or toxic (e.g. ethanol or certain chemotherapy regimens). Two low-grade insults appear to lead to greater overall severity than one single-site injury. In addition, the damage is greater than the expected additive effect.

Regional anesthesia has the potential to contribute to the double-crush syndrome. Causative factors may include mechanical needle trauma, ischemia from epinephrine-containing solutions or direct toxicity from local anesthetics. Hebl *et al.* (2006) found that 0.4% of patients with pre-existing neuropathy developed new or progressive neurologic defects after uneventful neuraxial anesthesia, a rate that is at least 10 times higher than that of the general population. However, peripheral nerve blocks may not carry the same risk: studies of axillary blocks (both single injection and catheters) for ulnar nerve transposition have shown a rate of neurologic complications no different from that of general anesthesia. This is especially telling because these patients by definition have pre-existing neuropathy and are having their nerves manipulated surgically, putting them at high risk. One explanation for the apparent difference in risk between neuraxial and peripheral nerve blockade might be the presence of the generous amount of connective tissue both surrounding and within the substance of the nerves in the axilla, compared to the relatively "raw" state of nerves in the intrathecal space, although this is hypothetical. Figure 13.6 illustrates the potential double-crush that has occurred in this case, with a subclinical traumatic injury (either via the original injury or the operative procedure) to the radial nerve, *plus* a more proximal insult at the brachial plexus level.

What is your course of action now?

When faced with a post-block neuropathy, it is essential to rule out immediately reversible causes first, such as vascular- or compression-related injuries. Other causes on the differential include a prolonged effect from an intraneural injection, nerve injury secondary to mechanical or chemical trauma (e.g. needle or local anesthetic) or the exacerbation of a pre-existing neuropathic condition. Fortunately, the vast majority of acute neuropathies resolve on their own. However, in some cases it is worth performing diagnostic testing to aid in determining prognosis. The algorithm for how to manage post-block neuropathy can be found in Chapter 19.

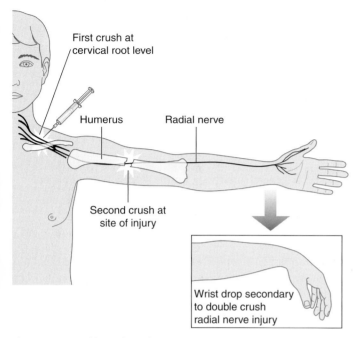

First crush at cervical root level

Humerus   Radial nerve

Second crush at site of injury

Wrist drop secondary to double crush radial nerve injury

Figure 13.6 Double-crush syndrome. A pre-existing subclinical peripheral nerve lesion (e.g. stretching or compression) is unmasked when a second insult (e.g. trauma or local anesthetic toxicity from a nerve block) is applied to the same nerve.

References and further reading

Bergman, B. D., Hebl, J. R., Kent, J., Horlocker, T. T. (2003). Neurologic complications of 405 consecutive continuous axillary catheters. *Anesthesia and Analgesia*, **96**, 247–52.

Borgeat, A., Aguirre, J., Curt, A. (2010). Case scenario: neurologic complication after continuous interscalene block. *Anesthesiology*, **112**, 742–5.

Childs, S. G. (2003). Double crush syndrome. *Orthopaedic Nursing / National Association of Orthopaedic Nurses*, **22**, 117–21.

Halaszynski, T. M. (2011). Ultrasound brachial plexus anesthesia and analgesia for upper extremity surgery: essentials of our current understanding, 2011. *Current Opinion in Anaesthesiology*, **24**, 581–91.

Hebl, J. R., Horlocker, T. T., Sorenson, E. J., Schroeder, D. R. (2001). Regional anesthesia does not increase the risk of postoperative neuropathy in patients undergoing ulnar nerve transposition. *Anesthesia and Analgesia*, **93**, 1606–11.

Hebl, J. R., Kopp, S. L., Schroeder, D. R., Horlocker, T. T. (2006). Neurologic complications after neuraxial anesthesia or analgesia in patients with preexisting peripheral sensorimotor neuropathy or diabetic polyneuropathy. *Anesthesia and Analgesia*, **103**, 1294–9.

Regional anesthesia for burns

Key aspects of case

1. Considerations for regional versus general anesthesia for the acutely burned patient.
2. Regional analgesia for dressing changes and excision and grafting procedures.

Case presentation

A 21-year-old woman is brought to hospital by ambulance after being involved in an explosion at a methamphetamine lab that she and her boyfriend operated out of their basement. She has what appear to be superficial and/or deep partial thickness burns to her anterior abdomen and lower chest, and her entire right forearm. She is resuscitated with crystalloid in the emergency room and transferred to the burn unit for management of her acute post-burn course. She is able to maintain her own airway and her oxygenation and ventilation are acceptable, with no evidence of inhalation injury. During her frequent dressing changes she complains of severe pain, which is inadequately treated with opioids. Moreover, she experiences several episodes of nausea and vomiting that are associated with the use of fentanyl for these painful procedures.

Case discussion

What are the priorities in the early management of burn injuries?

Approximately 10% of all burns present with additional traumatic injuries, reinforcing the need to adhere to basic principles of initial trauma resuscitation.

- **Airway:** a high index of suspicion must be maintained for inhalation injury. History of confinement in a burning environment or suggestive signs of inhalation injury (e.g. singed nasal hairs, carbonaceous sputum) should prompt consideration of *immediate intubation*. The orophaynx acts as a heat sink and can rapidly swell with edema, causing loss of the airway.

- **Breathing:** assume carbon monoxide (CO) exposure in patients burned in enclosed areas; administer high-flow 100% oxygen; follow arterial blood gases (ABGs) for carboxyhemoglobin levels.

- **Fluid resuscitation:** any burn with total body surface area (TBSA) >20% requires large-bore (+/− central) IV access and resuscitation with 2–4 ml/kg of a balanced salt solution for each 1% BSA affected by deep partial thickness and full thickness burns; in children, titrate fluid

Table 14.1 Classification of burns based on depth

Classification	Depth of burn	Signs and symptoms
First-degree	Epidermis only	Red, painful
Superficial partial thickness	Epidermis and papillary (superficial) dermis	Pink, painful blisters Heal 2–3 weeks
Deep partial thickness	Reticular (deep) dermis	Skin red and white Thick, often ruptured blisters Heal in 3–6 weeks
Full thickness	Full depth of dermis	White, leathery appearance Not painful Skin grafting necessary for healing

to maintain a urine output of 1 ml/kg/h. Respiratory burns represent a large area of increased vascular permeability and therefore an increased fluid requirement.

How are burn injuries assessed?

Body surface area is commonly calculated using the rule of nines: the head and arms are 9% each, the legs and anterior/posterior torso are 18% each, and the genitalia/perineum is 1%. Infants have proportionately larger heads (18%) and smaller legs (14%). The depth of burn is classified as shown in Table 14.1.

What are the characteristics of pain related to burns? How is burn pain treated?

Pain related to burn injuries can range from mild to debilitating, depending on the area involved and the depth of the burn. Skin nociceptors that are not destroyed transmit pain immediately after injury, and the perception of pain is complicated by both primary and secondary hyperalgesia, which occur at the wound and spinal level, respectively. Following resuscitation and admission, patients undergo a number of procedures, such as dressing changes, wound debridement, physiotherapy and skin grafting, each of which triggers a new cascade of painful impulses. This pattern of brief, intense painful procedures superimposed on moderate background pain makes effective analgesia challenging in these patients. Such procedures can occasionally be severe enough to require general anesthesia or deep sedation in the ICU or operating room. This is disadvantageous for a number of reasons, not the least of which is the frequent interruption of enteral nutrition to keep patients NPO at a time when their metabolic demand is supranormal.

Opioids remain the mainstay of pain management in the burn unit. While infusions of long-acting opioids are often required, short-acting and titratable opioids such as remifentanil can be ideal for brief, intense stimuli. Other adjuncts that have been used effectively include acetaminophen, intravenous lidocaine, ketamine, nitrous oxide, dexmedetomidine, gabapentin and amitriptyline. NSAIDs are commonly given, but must be used with caution in those patients with altered hemostasis and large areas to be grafted, as the platelet inhibition can lead to excessive bleeding. Topical local anesthetics have been advocated by some, but their use is limited by the size of the affected area (<25% BSA is recommended) and the potential for systemic toxicity.

What are the advantages and disadvantages to regional anesthesia in the burned patient?

There are several challenges to using regional analgesia in the burned patient. These patients are especially prone to infection owing to loss of the barrier function of the skin and an altered immune response. As such, percutaneous procedures such as nerve blocks should be chosen with care, particularly if an indwelling catheter is to be used. Catheters should not be placed through burned skin. Burns result in a hypercoagulable state, and deep blocks or neuraxial analgesic techniques are generally safe unless the patient develops coagulation abnormalities from sepsis or profound blood loss without factor replacement.

Because of the repetitive nature of the procedural pain in the burn unit, single injection techniques are not ideal. Continuous peripheral or neuraxial catheters provide the means to provide both background and incidental analgesia. The concentration of local anesthetic for background infusion is usually in the analgesic range (e.g. ropivacaine 0.2%, bupivacaine 0.125%). For severely painful procedures, boluses of short–intermediate-acting local anesthetics at higher concentrations provide ideal conditions (e.g. lidocaine 1.5–2%).

The advantages to avoiding deep sedation and general anesthesia for brief ICU procedures should be obvious and arc discussed elsewhere. Because these patients frequently require large doses of opioids, side effects such as nausea and vomiting, respiratory depression and constipation are frequent. Any technique that reduces reliance on these drugs should be encouraged. Much of the morbidity in burned patients relates to the profound stress response and the resultant effects on metabolism, wound healing and immune function. Neural blockade of a discretely burned area can substantially reduce the nociceptive input to the CNS, which may improve the overall recovery profile. For example, Pedersen *et al.* (1996) have shown that neural blockade reduces the incidence of hyperalgesia following thermal injury. For skin grafting procedures, regional analgesia results in reduced vasospasm and local thrombosis, effects that are deleterious to graft function.

On day 1 the patient complains of extreme pain with dressing changes to the chest, abdomen and forearm. You are consulted regarding possible regional analgesic options.

What are the options in this case?

For the burns on the anterior abdominal wall and inferior chest, practical choices are limited to an epidural technique or bilateral continuous paravertebral blockade. Intercostal blocks can be effective, but require multiple levels (↑risk of pneumothorax). Providing there are no contraindications to a neuraxial technique such as coagulopathy or local infection, it is probably simplest to place a thoracic epidural catheter. The insertion site should be chosen based on the estimated middle of the affected dermatomal distribution (probably about T6–7 in this case).

Choices are more extensive for analgesia of the forearm, as any brachial plexus approach could be utilized. For what might be a prolonged catheter technique, the infraclavicular approach has the advantage of improved patient comfort (versus interscalene) and is easily secured to the anterior chest wall with little mobile skin (versus axillary or supraclavicular).

Provided there is no locally injured skin in the lateral infraclavicular region, this would be a good choice.

On day 7 after the injury,the patient is deemed stable enough to be transferred to the operating room for excision of the burned skin and autologous grafting from the anterior thigh to the forearm. The epidural was removed on day 4.

You decide to add a femoral nerve catheter using ultrasound guidance. What are the technical tips for this?

The general principles of continuous femoral catheter placement are similar to a single injection femoral block.

- A linear transducer is placed on the inguinal crease in a transverse orientation and the femoral vessels and nerve are identified (see full description in Chapter 11).

- While a 50-mm Tuohy needle is often of sufficient length to reach the nerve from the surface, a longer needle (e.g. 10 cm) allows for a skin puncture several centimeters lateral to the transducer. This helps in two ways: (1) it creates a more shallow needle path to the nerve, rendering a better image of the needle on the ultrasound monitor; and (2) it results in a greater length of catheter under the skin, and, in particular, within sartorius and iliacus muscles. This decreases the likelihood of catheter displacement afterwards.

- Once the needle tip is adjacent to the nerve, a small (5–7 ml) bolus of local anesthetic is administered to "open up" the space and confirm correct placement. The transducer can then be set aside briefly while the catheter is advanced 1–2 cm beyond the tip of the needle (it is important to know in advance which markings on the catheter equate with catheter emergence through the needle tip as it is advanced).

- The needle is removed, and the femoral area imaged again with the transducer. Often the catheter cannot be visualized, but its position can be inferred by bolusing local anesthetic and observing the spread next to the nerve. The color Doppler function is also useful for this (Figure 14.1). Occasionally the catheter will have to be withdrawn several centimeters

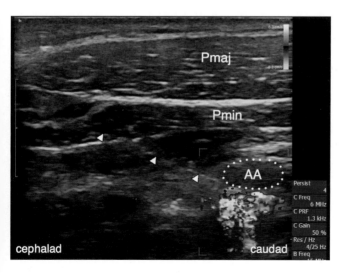

Figure 14.1 Catheter position following ultrasound-guided infraclavicular brachial plexus block. The catheter can be seen at various points along its course (arrowheads) but the tip is not well defined. Color Doppler is used to highlight its position, which in this case is deep to the axillary artery (AA). This should result in an effective block. Pmaj, Pectoralis major muscle; Pmin, pectoralis minor muscle.

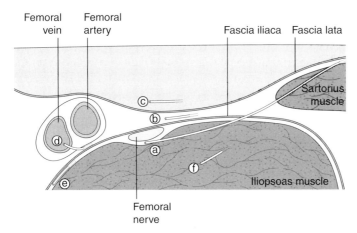

Femoral vein   Femoral artery   Fascia iliaca   Fascia lata

Sartorius muscle

Femoral nerve

Iliopsoas muscle

Figure 14.2 Possible femoral catheter tip locations. Correct placement adjacent to the nerve and deep to the fascia iliaca is represented by position (a). Positions (b) and (c) are superficial to the fascia iliaca and will result in a poor block, if any. Care must be taken not to push the catheter too far and into a vessel (d). Likewise, inattention to final catheter tip position can result in a failed block owing to excessive medial (e) or intramuscular (f) positioning.

as the tip was inadvertently placed too medially or too deep. It is recommended that the catheter be withdrawn 1 cm at a time, followed by a small bolus, so that the catheter is not displaced from the correct plane.

- It is critical for block success that the tip of the catheter lie beneath the fascia iliaca (Figure 14.2). There are multiple "wrong" places for the catheter tip to be, some of which are unsafe (e.g. in the vein) and some of which simply result in a failed block (e.g. subcutaneous), highlighting the need for visual confirmation of position using ultrasound.

- The catheter is secured and connected to an infusion pump programmed to infuse at 5 ml/h with a patient-controlled bolus of 5 ml every 30–45 minutes.

Are there particular risks to infusing local anesthetics through two peripheral nerve catheters in burn patients?

Peripheral nerve catheters are often used in combination, both for relief of distant injuries in trauma patients and to optimize lower extremity analgesia following elective surgery (e.g. femoral and sciatic catheters following total knee arthroplasty). The principal concern with continuous infusions of ropivacaine is systemic toxicity, although reported cases in the literature are rare. Multiple factors play a role in the likelihood of developing toxicity, including patient comorbidities (e.g. acidosis), technical errors (e.g. failure to aspirate) or relative degree of systemic absorption caused by vascularity at the site of administration (e.g. intercostal is high, sciatic is low).

Probably the best evidence of the safety of multiple catheters comes from the military experience. For example, Plunkett and Buckenmaier (2008) reported the case of a soldier who received infusions of ropivacaine 0.2% through three simultaneous catheters (bilateral sciatic plus a femoral catheter) continuously for 2 weeks. The patient received a total background infusion of 30 ml/h plus a further 10 ml every 30 minutes as required, and tolerated the therapy with no evidence of toxic symptoms or signs.

When ropivacaine is administered intravenously, the threshold for detecting neurologic symptoms has been estimated to be approximately 2.2 mcg/ml (total) and 0.15 mcg/ml (unbound fraction). In the above report, the total plasma ropivacaine drawn at 24 h following the initiation of the infusion was measured at 5.792 mcg/ml, while the unbound fraction was <0.1 mcg/ml. It is likely the unbound fraction that is responsible for the few cases of toxicity following large doses and/or continuous infusions. Alpha-1 acid glycoprotein (AAG) is the plasma protein that binds local anesthetics. As an acute phase reactant, levels of AAG are known to be significantly elevated in burns (and trauma in general), an effect that lasts at least 20 days. This may provide an increased margin of safety during large infusions in these patients.

Practically speaking, it is difficult to measure ropivacaine levels, and so judgments on the appropriateness and/or duration of multiple catheters should be made taking all of the above factors into consideration. One additional way to potentially increase the safety margin of multiple catheters is to reduce the background infusion rate and rely more (or completely) on the bolus function. For example, a femoral catheter bolused with 10–12 ml of 0.2% ropivacaine should provide analgesia for at least 4–6 h, effectively reducing the dose over that time period by 40–50 ml.

References and further reading

Bleckner, L. L., Bina, S., Kwon, K. H. *et al.* (2010). Serum ropivacaine concentrations and systemic local anesthetic toxicity in trauma patients receiving long-term continuous peripheral nerve block catheters. *Anesthesia and Analgesia*, **110**, 630–4.

Cuignet, O., Pirson, J., Boughrouph, J., Duville, D. (2004). The efficacy of continuous fascia iliaca compartment block for pain management in burn patients undergoing skin grafting procedures. *Anesthesia and Analgesia*, **98**, 1077–81.

Dadure, C., Acosta, C., Capdevila, X. (2004). Perioperative pain management of a complex orthopedic surgical procedure with double continuous nerve blocks in a burned child. *Anesthesia and Analgesia*, **98**, 1653–5.

Gupta, A., Bhandari, P. S., Shrivastava, P. (2007). A study of regional nerve blocks and local anesthetic creams (Prilox) for donor sites in burn patients. *Burns: Journal of the International Society for Burn Injuries*, **33**, 87–91.

Karacalar, A., Karacalar, S., Uçkunkaya, N., Sahin, S., Ozcan, B. (1998). Combined use of axillary block and lateral femoral cutaneous nerve block in upper-extremity injuries requiring large skin grafts. *The Journal of Hand Surgery*, **23**, 1100–5.

Pedersen, J. L., Crawford, M. E., Dahl, J. B., Brennan, J., Kehlet, H. (1996). Effect of preemptive nerve block on inflammation and hyperalgesia after human thermal injury. *Anesthesiology*, **84**, 1020–6.

Plunkett, A. R., Buckenmaier, C. C., 3rd. (2008). Safety of multiple, simultaneous continuous peripheral nerve block catheters in a patient receiving therapeutic low-molecular-weight heparin. *Pain Medicine (Malden, Mass.)*, **9**, 624–7.

Richardson, P., Mustard, L. (2009). The management of pain in the burns unit. *Burns: Journal of the International Society for Burn Injuries*, **35**, 921–36.

Chapter 15

Regional anesthesia, penetrating abdominal trauma and sepsis

Key aspects of case

1. Role of epidural anesthesia/analgesia and rectus sheath blockade for exploratory laparotomy following penetrating trauma.

2. Abdominal compartment syndrome.

3. Management of an epidural catheter in the septic patient.

Case presentation

A 22-year-old male sustains a gunshot wound to the abdomen following an argument with a neighbor. His vitals on arrival to hospital are BP 135/87, HR 106 bpm, RR 24, T 36.5°C and SpO₂ 100% on facemask. He is maintaining his airway and has no other obvious injuries. He denies any medical history but admits to regular heroin use. The bullet trajectory appears to be tangential through the abdominal cavity, entering through the left anterolateral abdominal wall and exiting through the right side. He is taken urgently to the operating room, where he undergoes an exploratory laparotomy under general anesthesia. The bullet is found to have perforated the descending colon and small bowel, both of which are repaired primarily. Blood loss throughout the operation was 900 ml, and the patient was resuscitated with 5 l of crystalloid. He is extubated uneventfully and transferred to the ICU, where he complains of severe pain in his abdomen, despite a total of 3 mg of hydromorphone in the last hour.

Case discussion

What are the regional analgesic options for pain management following abdominal trauma?

The abdominal wall is innervated by the anterior primary rami of T7–L1. These nerves emerge from their respective intervertebral foraminae and travel between the second and third muscle layer in both the thorax (internal and innermost intercostal) and abdomen (internal oblique and transversus abdominis) before terminating in the midline. Regional blocks can be performed effectively at most points along their course (Table 15.1).

What are the pitfalls of epidural analgesia in abdominal trauma?

- **Coagulopathy**: a rare but devastating complication of epidural analgesia is spinal hematoma. Its true incidence is unknown; recent estimates place it at 1:150 000 following

Table 15.1 Regional analgesic options for trauma to the abdominal wall

Approach	Advantages	Disadvantages	Distribution
Thoracic epidural analgesia (TEA)	Gold standard block for abdomen Bilateral Titratable to desired level Contraindicated if coagulopathy, hypovolemia or unresponsive patient	Contraindicated if coagulopathy, severe hypovolemia (e.g. many trauma patients) Controversial in unconscious patients (possible ↑risk of neural damage with no ability to warn)	
Paravertebral	Excellent unilateral *or* bilateral block Less hypotension than epidural Can be safely performed in patients with bleeding diatheses or unconscious patients Titratable to desired level if catheter technique used	Two (versus one) catheters must be placed in order to achieve bilateral block If single injection technique used, *multiple* injections (e.g. 5–10 or more) required depending on one versus two sides, number of dermatomes desired, etc.	
Transversus abdominis plane (TAP) block	May provide mild–moderate pain control for some abdominal procedures Continuous catheter technique possible Can be safely performed in patients with bleeding diatheses or unconscious patients No concern re: hypotension	Area of coverage variable and depends on approach (i.e. subcostal versus suprailiac, etc.). The commonly described approach (between iliac crest and costal margin) may not provide anesthesia	
Rectus sheath block	Good pain control for periumbilical and moderate length midline incisions Relatively safe, especially if performed with ultrasound No concerns re: unconscious patients, hypotension.	Smaller area of analgesia compared to other abdominal blocks	

epidural anesthesia, but these data were largely collected in the era prior to the routine use of perioperative thromboprophylaxis (e.g. low molecular weight heparin). Trauma patients are frequently coagulopathic from hypothermia and/or massive blood loss, and may go on to develop worsening hemostasis from liver injury or hypoperfusion, sepsis or disseminated intravascular coagulation. Guidelines from both North America and Europe suggest avoiding the placement or removal of epidural catheters with INR >1.5.

- **Hypotension**: epidural local anesthetics (LAs) cause sympatholysis and the greater the infused volume/rate, the greater the expected degree of arterial hypotension. This can often be mitigated with the use of vasopressors, but epidural analgesia should be used with caution in patients who are hypovolemic or under-resuscitated.

- **Neurologic impairment**: conventional wisdom suggests that epidural catheters should not be inserted in patients who are unconscious or cannot respond appropriately, for fear of unknowingly causing spinal cord damage. This is a controversial assertion, as the ability of an awake patient to report paresthesias in the event of needle/cord contact is not 100% (see Chapter 17). However, most clinicians in a trauma setting will wait until the patient can communicate prior to placing an epidural. Thoracic epidural analgesia (TEA) should be avoided in patients with head injury or lumbar spine injury, as it complicates neurologic evaluation.

The postoperative blood work shows a hemoglobin of 9.5 mg/dl and normal prothrombin time (PT) and partial thromboplastin time (PTT). You decide to place an epidural for analgesia.

Where should the epidural be placed? What medications should be infused?

The insertion point of an epidural should always match the incision. In this case, the midline laparotomy extends above and below the umbilicus for several centimeters. An insertion point of T9–10 is therefore best, as it will result in a discrete band of analgesia at just the required dermatomes, while sparing the lower lumbar and sacral dermatomes. Patients with thoracic epidurals can often still have use of their legs, and can avoid prolonged urinary catheterization as retention caused by sacral blockade is avoided.

The goal here is analgesia, not anesthesia. As with all regional techniques, the lowest effective concentration of LA should be used. Ropivacaine 0.2% or bupivacaine 0.125% are good choices. The addition of fentanyl 4 mcg/ml provides an increase in the quality of analgesia and reduces the overall amount of LA required.

Following placement of the epidural, the patient appears more comfortable. However, 16 hours later the patient's condition deteriorates, with a decrease in his urine output and progressive respiratory difficulty over 2 hours.

What is abdominal compartment syndrome (ACS)?

ACS refers to organ dysfunction caused by intra-abdominal hyptertension. It is most commonly diagnosed in trauma patients, with an incidence of 1–15%. Intra-abdominal pressure (IAP) is usually 5–7 mmHg, and is considered abnormal if >12 mmHg. Above that threshold, abdominal perfusion begins to suffer, and organ dysfunction ensues, particularly of the gut, kidneys and liver. The increased IAP also results in reduced venous return, cardiac output and alveolar ventilation, which combine to worsen perfusion and acidosis.

Intracranial pressure is frequently elevated in ACS, and the reduced intra-abdominal compliance often results in wound complications.

Diagnosis relies on the measurement of IAP, as physical exam is insensitive and imaging studies are also unhelpful. This is typically done by transducing the aspiration port of a clamped and saline-infused Foley catheter. Treatment consists of the following in a step-wise fashion as dictated by IAP and/or organ dysfunction.

1. Evacuate intraluminal contents (nasogastric/rectal tube, enemas, stop enteral feeding).
2. Evacuate intra-abdominal space-occupying lesions (e.g. percutaneous drainage).
3. Improve abdominal wall compliance (sedation/anesthesia/neuromuscular blockade, consider reverse Trendelenburg position).
4. Optimize fluid administration (goal: zero to negative fluid balance; also consider hypertonic saline, ultrafiltration).
5. Optimize tissue perfusion (goal-directed fluid resuscitation → fluids/vasopressors to keep abdominal perfusion pressure [mean arterial pressure (MAP)–IAP] >60 mmHg).
6. Consider surgical decompression and temporary abdominal wall closure if IAP >20 mmHg and refractory to medical management.

The patient is found to have an IAP of 23 mmHg. He is taken to the operating room and a decompressive laparotomy is performed.

Should the epidural be used as part of the anesthetic?

No. Morbidity and mortality related to ACS is proportional to the degree of hypoperfusion of various organs. The inevitable sympathectomy associated with a thoracic epidural will further decrease arterial pressure, thereby decreasing abdominal perfusion pressure. This patient is also suffering from respiratory impairment and requires endotracheal intubation, so the benefit gained from continued epidural analgesia is minimal.

What are the anatomical considerations regarding the rectus sheath block? Can rectus sheath catheters be placed prior to closure of the abdomen?

- The rectus sheath encompasses the rectus abdominis muscles and contains the anterior rami of the lower six thoracic nerves (T7–12). It is formed by the aponeuroses of the three lateral abdominal muscles, the external oblique, the internal oblique and the transversus abdominis (Figure 15.1).
- Below the arcuate line (located at approximately the level of the anterior superior iliac spine), the posterior wall of the rectus sheath is deficient, as all three aponeurotic layers travel anterior to the rectus muscles.
- Each of the nerves enters the rectus sheath from the lateral side and travels deep to the muscle before turning anteriorly and puncturing the anterior wall of the sheath to supply the skin of the central abdomen. Rectus sheath blockade involves the administration of LA deep to the rectus muscle on each side within the sheath. This block provides excellent analgesia for procedures about the midline, but does not extend lateral to the linea semilunaris (the lateral border of the rectus abdominis muscles).

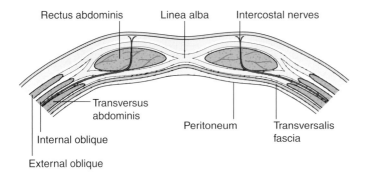

Figure 15.1 Transverse section of the anterior abdominal wall showing the rectus abdominis musculature and the intercostal nerves that travel through it.

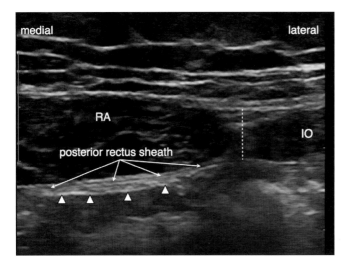

Figure 15.2 Sonoanatomy relevant to the rectus sheath block. The rectus sheath envelopes the rectus abdominis muscle (RA) and creates a potential space immediately deep to the posterior wall of the muscle belly. Care must be taken not to puncture the sheath, as the peritoneum (arrowheads) is in close proximity. Lateral to the RA can be seen the aponeurosis of the lateral muscles of the abdominal wall (dotted line) and the internal oblique muscle (IO).

- Ultrasonography has made rectus sheath blocks quite safe and easy. The transducer is placed just lateral to the umbilicus and the rectus abdominis muscle within the sheath is located (Figure 15.2). Color Doppler should always be used to identify the inferior epigastric artery which travels within the sheath to avoid puncture.

- A short beveled needle is then advanced either in-plane or out-of-plane through the rectus muscle. As the needle approaches the posterior wall of the sheath, intermittent small boluses of injectate should be delivered to confirm needletip location (the peritoneum lies directly below the posterior sheath).

- After negative aspiration, 20 ml of LA per side is administered, which should result in blockade of T8–T12. Ropivacaine 0.2% or bupivacaine or levobupivacaine 0.125% are good choices.

- Alternatively, catheters can be placed using a standard epidural catheter kit or peripheral nerve catheter kit. Once correct needletip position is ensured, 5 ml of LA is administered and the catheter advanced 1–2 cm beyond the tip of the needle. After negative aspiration,

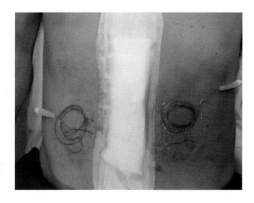

Figure 15.3 Patient with bilateral rectus sheath catheters following midline laparotomy.

the tip position is confirmed by visualization of additional spread with injection on ultrasound. The catheters are secured, connected to infusion pumps programmed to infuse at 8–10 ml/h (for each side) (Figure 15.3).

- Rectus sheath catheters can also be placed by the surgeon prior to closure using the same needle and catheter kit. By palpating the posterior sheath from within the abdomen, the needle is directed percutaneously to the plane just superficial to his/her fingers, and the catheter advanced.

The patient returns to the ICU intubated but his condition continues to worsen. On POD#3 his heart rate is 112 bpm, BP 89/48 mmHg and his temperature is 39.2°C. Lab work shows an elevated PT (INR 1.9) and lactate level, decreased platelets and fibrinogen and the presence of D-dimers. The epidural catheter remains in place, but has not been used since the diagnosis of ACS.

What impact does epidural anesthesia/analgesia have on outcome in septic patients?

The benefit of epidural anesthesia in sepsis remains unknown. While the idea of providing a sympathectomy and increasing cardiac index is theoretically attractive, little human data is available, and the animal data is somewhat contradictory. In one septic rat model, TEA had a beneficial effect on pulmonary endothelial integrity in the hyperdynamic phase of sepsis, but not in the hypodynamic (late) sepsis. Two recent studies in sheep with endotoxemia suggest that TEA is safe and may improve renal perfusion. However, numerous other studies either fail to show a benefit or, in fact, demonstrate worsened mortality with TEA in sepsis.

One concern in this setting is the risk for epidural abscess. When queried about a hypothetical patient with a bowel perforation who had a fever and an elevated white blood cell count, but was hemodynamically stable, only 27% of UK anesthesiologists would perform an epidural for analgesia. The most common reason for avoidance was fear of epidural abscess, although the risk of systemic sepsis on this complication is unknown. The most common organism causing epidural abscesses is *Staphylococcus aureus*. The risk of developing a spinal abscess related to Gram-negative sepsis may for this reason be quite small. On the other hand, the benefit to the pulmonary system of epidural analgesia is well documented, and the risk–benefit analysis must be performed for each individual patient. For example, TEA is used frequently and safely for decortication of empyema, and often permits early extubation in a population at risk for prolonged mechanical ventilation.

What should be done regarding the removal of the catheter in this patient with disseminated intravascular coagulation?

While epidural techniques are contraindicated in coagulopathy a priori, occasionally impaired hemostasis occurs while a catheter is *in situ*. The dilemma in this patient is whether to wait for removal until the coagulopathy resolves (but increasing the risk of epidural abscess or catheter migration into a vessel) or whether to proceed with prompt removal. Cases have been reported of epidural catheter removal after systemic anticoagulation resulting in spinal hematomas. However, since the catheter is no longer useful, as a LA block would confuse the diagnosis of spinal hematoma, the optimum balanced strategy is to remove it. The risk of epidural abscess increases directly with duration of catheterization, as does the risk of migration into an epidural vein, which can be a source of spinal bleeding, and these probably outweigh the relatively small risk of spinal hematoma from catheter removal.

Catheter removal may be preceded by the administration of plasma and/or cryoprecipitate so that coagulation factors and fibrinogen, respectively, are transiently replenished. Following removal, the patient should have neurologic examinations frequently (e.g. every 2 h) for the first 24 h, and the threshold for obtaining spinal imaging should be low. Clearly, neurologic assessment is difficult in the intubated and/or unconscious patient; in these cases, delayed removal may be advisable until such time as the patient can cooperate with motor examination. Should the patient at any time show evidence of lower extremity neurologic deterioration, an immediate spinal MRI should be performed and a neurosurgeon consulted for evaluation and possible decompressive laminectomy.

Further reading

Balogh, Z. J., van Wessem, K., Yoshino, O., Moore, F. A. (2009). Postinjury abdominal compartment syndrome: are we winning the battle? *World Journal of Surgery*, **33**, 1134–41.

Daudel, F., Bone, H.-G., Traber, D. L. *et al.* (2006). Effects of thoracic epidural anesthesia on hemodynamics and global oxygen transport in ovine endotoxemia. *Shock (Augusta, Ga.)*, **26**, 615–19.

Daudel, F., Ertmer, C., Stubbe, H. D. *et al.* (2007). Hemodynamic effects of thoracic epidural analgesia in ovine hyperdynamic endotoxemia. *Regional Anesthesia and Pain Medicine*, **32**, 311–16.

Kotzé, A., Hinton, W., Crabbe, D. C. G., Carrigan, B. J. (2007). Audit of epidural analgesia in children undergoing thoracotomy for decortication of empyema. *British Journal of Anaesthesia*, **98**, 662–6.

Mutz, C., Vagts, D. A. (2009). Thoracic epidural anesthesia in sepsis – is it harmful or protective? *Critical Care (London, England)*, **13**, 182.

Nightingale, J. J., Burmeister, L., Hopkins, D. (2011). A national survey of the use of epidural analgesia in patients with sepsis undergoing laparotomy. *Anaesthesia*, **66**, 311–12.

Rizoli, S., Mamtani, A., Scarpelini, S., Kirkpatrick, A. W. (2010). Abdominal compartment syndrome in trauma resuscitation. *Current Opinion in Anaesthesiology*, **23**, 251–7.

Sprung, J., Cheng, E. Y., Patel, S. (1992). When to remove an epidural catheter in a parturient with disseminated intravascular coagulation. *Regional Anesthesia*, **17**, 351–4.

Regional anesthesia in the injured obese patient

Key aspects of case

1. Considerations for regional anesthesia in obesity.
2. The use of regional anesthesia in the setting of the very difficult airway.

Case presentation

A 43-year-old female is brought to hospital by ambulance following a head-on motor vehicle accident (MVA) in which she was the driver. She was not wearing a seatbelt, but airbags were deployed. Injuries consist of a mild concussion, abrasions to her face and forehead, two hairline rib fractures on the right side and what appears to be a posterior dislocation of her right hip. Her vitals are currently stable, and she appears to have no life-threatening or other serious injuries, although she is complaining of severe pain in her right hip and pelvis. She is obese, with a weight and height of 115 kg (253 lbs) and 160 cm (63 inches), respectively. Her body mass index (BMI) is 42 kg/m². She has a short, thick neck with limited range of motion. Her mouth opening is limited, and she has a Mallampati score of IV on airway examination; she is wearing a semi-rigid cervical collar. Her medical history is positive for obstructive sleep apnea (OSA) and hypertension. After initial evaluation and stabilization, the plan is to perform a closed reduction of her hip in the emergency room.

Case discussion

What are the considerations for management of trauma in the obese population?

Obesity is a risk factor for trauma: the morbidly obese are 50% more likely to suffer non-fatal unintentional injury requiring medical attention. They are at higher risk for MVAs, presumably because of an increased incidence of OSA, which carries a sevenfold increased risk of traffic accidents. The altered body habitus in the obese leads to different patterns of injury. For example, obese patients injured in MVAs have less severe abdominal injuries (owing to a "cushioning effect"), but higher injury severity of lower extremity injuries. The severity of head injury following MVA is probably no greater, and some studies show it is reduced in obesity, for reasons that are not known. Morbid obesity is an independent risk factor for mortality and pulmonary complications following severe trauma.

Practical issues may occur in prehospital transport of obese injured patients, including difficulties with extrication, splinting or immobilization of the cervical spine due to size. Similarly, obesity can hamper diagnosis based on subtle physical findings such as breath or heart sounds, make ultrasound (i.e. FAST scan) evaluation difficult, and preclude some diagnostic modalities such as CT scanning.

The airway is always a consideration in obese patients, and the presence of a reduced functional residual capacity predisposes to early hypoxemia. The high rate of OSA in this population also puts them at risk for obstruction and desaturation during sleep as well as sedation.

Before the hip is reduced, what other information is required?

Posterior hip dislocation is an infrequently seen injury, but almost always occurs as a result of femoral axial loading (e.g. impact between the knee and the dashboard in an MVA). Because of the high-energy nature of posterior hip dislocation, a full trauma evaluation is mandated to rule out other injuries. Associated orthopedic injuries include ipsilateral femoral neck or shaft fractures, pelvic fractures, knee fracture and/or dislocation, and spinal fractures. A careful neurovascular examination is required because of the risk of injury to the sciatic nerve and/or femoral/popliteal vasculature. If there is an associated femoral neck or hip fracture, open or closed reduction in the operating room should be performed; otherwise, prompt closed reduction of the femoral head is warranted to reduce the risk of osteonecrosis.

Due to her obesity and the anticipated difficult airway, your preference is to avoid sedation and/or general anesthesia.

Can this be done under regional anesthesia? What nerves need to be blocked to provide anesthesia to the hip joint?

Closed reduction of dislocated hips is often attempted with sedation. However, frequently pain, inadequate muscle relaxation and/or patient concerns regarding deep sedation (e.g. increased intracranial pressure, OSA) make sedation a less than ideal choice. Regional anesthesia can provide good analgesic conditions and appropriate muscle relaxation without the risks of profound sedation.

The hip is supplied primarily by the branches of the lumbar plexus (femoral and obturator nerves). In addition, some articular branches arise from the sacral plexus, namely the superior gluteal nerve, the nerve to quadratus femoris, as well as directly from the sciatic nerve.

What are the regional anesthetic options available for this procedure?

Neuraxial anesthesia (either spinal or epidural) would provide excellent conditions for closed reduction. Since this is usually a brief procedure, a short-acting agent is preferred. Spinal block with 45 mg of chloroprocaine or epidural with 10–15 ml of 2% lidocaine are both acceptable choices, although there is little to be lost by using a longer-acting agent if choice is limited. Volumes should be carefully considered in the event that epidural anesthesia is chosen, as this increases the risk of local anesthetic systemic toxicity (LAST), which would require the *emergent* management of this patient's unfavorable airway.

Peripheral nerve block also requires the administration of greater volumes of local anesthetic (LA), and the risk of LAST should be weighed into the decision. Blockade of the lumbar plexus (i.e. femoral and obturator nerves) is all that is required for closed hip reduction and, although the addition of a proximal sciatic nerve block would provide complete anesthesia to the joint, it is unnecessary. The lumbar plexus can be approached either as two separate blocks of the femoral and obturator nerves, respectively, or via the posterior approach as a single injection.

How does the patient's body habitus impact your choice of technique?

Regional anesthesia has been shown to be more difficult in obese patients. Nielsen *et al.* (2005) showed that a BMI of >30 kg/m^2 was associated with a 1.62-fold increase in block failure. Practical considerations include access to the skin puncture site (e.g. the need for retraction of the pannus for femoral and/or obturator blocks), the requirement for longer than normal needles, difficulty with bony landmarks owing to increased subcutaneous adiposity and difficulty with ultrasound imaging.

Despite large rolls of abdominal fat in the morbidly obese, the spinal midline is often not as affected and neuraxial anesthesia can be surprisingly easy. Posterior lumbar plexus block can be more challenging because of the difficulty in estimating the depth to the transverse processes. Femoral and especially obturator blockade are challenging in those patients with large abdominal pannuses; the use of wide silk tape to retract the pannus helps in exposing the inguinal region, although ultrasound imaging of the specific nerves can still be difficult.

Should regional anesthesia be avoided in patients with a difficult airway?

Analysis of closed claims databases clearly shows that airway problems are the leading cause of anesthesia-related deaths. However, regional anesthesia in a patient with a difficult airway does not necessarily mean the airway is no longer an issue. There are multiple reports of well-intentioned regional anesthetics that resulted in a seizure, cardiac arrest or other event that resulted in the unsuccessful emergent management of a difficult airway.

Foley (2011) suggested that several factors should be weighed into the risk–benefit equation, including the expertise of the clinician (both at regional anesthesia and airway management), the cooperativeness of the patient, the cooperativeness of the surgeon to stop and permit an alternative technique if plan A fails, and the position of the patient during the procedure (i.e. airway access).

You decide that a short-acting spinal would be your first choice, but the patient refuses to undergo any neuraxial technique. After consideration of the pros and cons, you elect to perform a posterior lumbar plexus block.

What are the anatomical and technical considerations for this technique?

- The lumbar plexus originates from the spinal roots of L1–L4, with a contribution from T12. After the nerves emerge from the intervertebral foramina, they divide into anterior

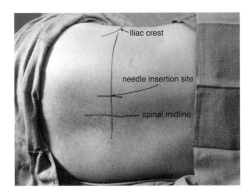

Figure 16.1 Landmarks for the lumbar plexus block. The needle insertion site is 4 cm lateral to the intersection of the midline and the intercristal line.

and posterior branches. The small posterior branches supply the skin of the lower back and paravertebral muscles. The anterior branches form the lumbar plexus within the substance of the psoas muscle, and emerge from the muscle as individual nerves in the pelvis. The clinically most important branches of the lumbar plexus are the femoral, obturator and lateral femoral cutaneous nerves, but the plexus also gives rise to the iliohypogastric, ilioinguinal and genitofemoral nerves.

- The patient is placed in the lateral decubitus position with a slight forward tilt. The clinician should assume a position from which the anterior thigh can be seen so that contractions of the quadriceps muscle are visible. The needle insertion site can be determined by: (1) palpating the iliac crest and drawing a transverse line extending to the midline; (2) palpating the midline; and (3) marking a point 4 cm lateral to the intersection of the first line and the midline of the back (Figure 16.1).

- After skin preparation and local infiltration, a 100-mm stimulating needle is inserted perpendicular to the skin (noting that the patient is tilted slightly away). The nerve stimulator should be set initially to deliver a current of 1.0 mA. As the needle is advanced, local twitches of the paravertebral muscles are first obtained at a depth of a few centimeters. The needle is then advanced further until twitches of the quadriceps muscle are obtained (usually at a depth of 6–8 cm). After these twitches are observed, the current should be lowered to produce stimulation between 0.2 and 0.5 mA. Following negative aspiration, 20–30 ml of LA are slowly injected. The volume of LA is usually determined by the goal: analgesia usually only requires 20 ml, whereas surgical anesthesia of the lower limb usually requires 30 ml.

- If the needle is advanced 8–10 cm without twitches, it should be withdrawn to skin, directed 5° medially and reinserted slowly. If this does not result in a motor response, the needle should be withdrawn completely, and a new skin insertion site made 1 cm closer to the midline, advancing perpendicular to the skin. It is important to avoid directing the needle in too medial a fashion, as this may result in epidural or subarachnoid block.

- If contact with the transverse process is made, the needle should be withdrawn several centimeters, redirected 10° cephalad or caudad, and reinserted to pass above or below the transverse process. The plexus lies 1.5–2 cm beyond the transverse process in most adults.

The block is performed with 25 ml of 0.375% ropivacaine and, within 10 minutes, the patient's pain is much improved. Despite this, the orthopedic surgeons are unable to reduce her hip, and instead plan to perform the procedure in the operating room with "more profound anesthesia."

You are still in favor of regional anesthesia and, after further discussion, the patient consents to a spinal anesthetic. Her surface anatomy is not helpful with respect to landmarking for the procedure.

How can ultrasound help?

There are two ways in which ultrasonography can be utilized with respect to neuraxial blocks. The first is as a pre-procedure scanning modality, to characterize the anatomy prior to a traditional "blind" technique. At present this remains the most popular use of the technology for the neuraxial indication. The other, more challenging, use is to facilitate real-time guidance of needles into the spinal space. Ultrasound imaging of the spine in obese patients is not always straightforward, but with practice it can become a very useful tool.

For practical purposes, the spinal column can be imaged in two primary planes. The paramedian oblique orientation (Figure 16.2) is useful for gaining a window to the dura, ligamentum flavum and spinal canal via the intervertebral foramina (Figure 16.3), and for determining the spinal level. The midline transverse orientation (Figure 16.4) is useful for determining the true midline, the midline depth to the ligamentum flavum and posterior

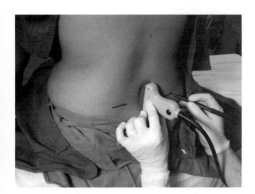

Figure 16.2 Paramedian oblique orientation for lumbar epidural scanning with a convex ultrasound transducer. The transducer is 1–2 cm off the midline, aimed towards the interlaminar foramina. Once a suitable level is found, it can be marked on the skin precisely.

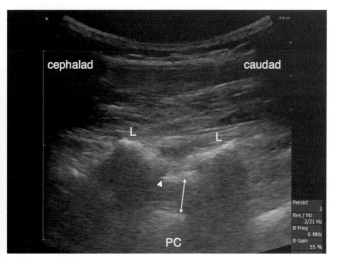

Figure 16.3 Sonoanatomy of the lumbar epidural region using the paramedian oblique view. The laminae of two adjacent vertebrae are seen, along with the "window" into the spinal canal (double-headed arrow). The dura (arrowhead) is seen easily, as is the posterior dura and vertebral body complex (PC).

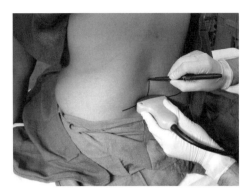

Figure 16.4 Transverse orientation for lumbar epidural scanning with a convex ultrasound transducer. This orientation allows for estimation of both depth and midline. The midline is being marked on the skin.

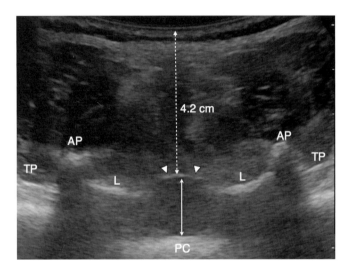

Figure 16.5 Sonoanatomy of the lumbar epidural region using the transverse view. The dura (arrowheads) is readily seen situated between two laminae (L). The spinal canal (double-headed arrow) is visualized between the dura and the posterior complex (PC). Other bony features include the articular processes (AP) and transverse processes (TP). Once the image is frozen, calipers can be used to measure the distance from the skin to the dura.

dura (also known together as the posterior complex), and for establishing the presence of any rotational defects (Figure 16.5). For both of these, it is critical to establish an acoustic window through non-bony structures to visualize the relevant structures such as the posterior complex and the spinal canal. In the transverse orientation, this often requires subtle cephalocaudad translation of the transducer with or without a slight cephalad tilt to avoid the beam impacting the spinous processes.

Once the spinal level is determined, a mark can be made on the skin just lateral to the probe. Similarly, a midline mark can be made during transverse imaging of the spine. The depth to the ligamentum can also be noted in either view by freezing the image and using the electronic calipers. The probe can then be removed and the two lines extended until they intersect, which should provide a useful needle insertion site.

References and further reading

Chin, K. J., Perlas, A. (2011). Ultrasonography of the lumbar spine for neuraxial and lumbar plexus blocks. *Current Opinion in Anaesthesiology*, **24**, 567–72.

Desapriya, E., Giulia, S., Subzwari, S., *et al.* (2011). Does obesity increase the risk of injury or mortality in motor vehicle crashes? A systematic review and meta-analysis.

Asia-Pacific Journal of Public Health/Asia-Pacific Academic Consortium for Public Health. [ePub ahead of print]

Evans, D. C., Stawicki, S. P. A., Davido, H. T., Eiferman, D. (2011). Obesity in trauma patients: correlations of body mass index with outcomes, injury patterns, and complications. *The American Surgeon*, 77, 1003–8.

Foley L. Airway management of patients with a history of difficult intubation for a peripheral procedure. In: Hung, O., Murphy, M. (2011). *Management of the Difficult and Failed Airway*, 2nd edn. New York: McGraw-Hill Professional.

Meroz, Y., Gozal, Y. (2007). Management of the obese trauma patient. *Anesthesiology Clinics*, 25, 91–8.

Nielsen, K. C., Guller, U., Steele, S. M. *et al.* (2005). Influence of obesity on surgical regional anesthesia in the ambulatory setting: an analysis of 9,038 blocks. *Anesthesiology*, 102, 181–7.

Sheth, M., Liles, C. H., Phillips, W. J., Lerant, A. (2008). Lumbar plexus block via a femoral approach for total hip arthroplasty dislocation reduction: a report of 2 cases. *European Journal of Emergency Medicine: Official Journal of the European Society for Emergency Medicine*, 15, 226–30.

Sifri, Z. C., Kim, H., Lavery, R., Mohr, A., Livingston, D. H. (2008). The impact of obesity on the outcome of emergency intubation in trauma patients. *The Journal of Trauma*, 65, 396–400.

Regional anesthesia and lower extremity trauma

Key aspects of case

1. The role of peripheral nerve blocks in anesthetized patients.
2. The role of various lower limb nerve blocks for ankle surgery.

Case presentation

A 33-year-old male presents to the emergency room after sustaining bilateral open calcaneal fractures. On history, he reports jumping out of a second floor bedroom window and landing on his feet before collapsing to the pavement. He was wearing only a bathrobe at the time, and was not wearing footwear. Upon initial evaluation, he is maintaining his airway and had no obvious cardiorespiratory injuries. He is complaining of severe pain in both ankles as well as his lower back and right shoulder. Further evaluation reveals a right anterior shoulder dislocation as well as a burst fracture of the L2 vertebral body. A gross neurologic examination is normal and CT imaging shows no spinal canal compromise. External blood loss has been minimal. Past medical history includes gout, but he has no allergies and takes only allopurinol. His last meal was 5 h ago. Vitals are BP 161/92 mmHg, HR 112 bpm, RR 24/min, T 36.7°C and SpO$_2$ 100% on facemask oxygen. He is scheduled to proceed to the operating room for open reduction internal fixation (ORIF) of the bilateral ankle fractures and closed reduction of the shoulder dislocation.

Case discussion

What are the key issues in the management of calcaneal fractures?

Acute traumatic calcaneal fractures are usually seen in young patients who have sustained a fall from a height, typically >2 m. These injuries are bilateral in 10% of cases. Because the mechanism of injury involves an axial load, there is concomitant lumbar or thoracic spinal injury in 5–15% of patients, most frequently at the thoracolumbar junction (i.e. T11, T12, L1 or L2). There are usually no other injuries. The choice of operative versus non-operative therapy is controversial, except in the setting of open fractures, and many closed fractures are treated conservatively.

What are the anesthetic options for this case?

There are two limiting factors to this case. First, there are planned procedures on two distant sites, the ankles and the shoulder, and thus two sources of procedural pain. Second, there is a lumbar vertebral injury that effectively precludes the use of neuraxial anesthesia. While it is theoretically possible to perform three separate nerve blocks (e.g. bilateral sciatic blocks plus an interscalene block), this is impractical and may put the patient at risk for local anesthetic toxicity. In addition, this patient is suffering from lower back pain due to the fracture and would likely not tolerate "block plus sedation." General anesthesia appears to be the best option for surgical anesthesia.

What are the options for postoperative analgesia?

This patient should receive multimodal analgesia with acetaminophen, NSAIDs and/or COX-2 inhibitors unless contraindicated. Because his pain will be multifocal (lumbar spine, shoulder and bilateral ankles), intravenous patient-controlled opioid analgesia should be prescribed. However, an opportunity exists to reduce his pain burden substantially by performing bilateral peripheral nerve blockade of the lower limbs. The maximum duration of a single shot block is 18–24 h; a continuous catheter, on the other hand, will allow for several days of pain relief.

What is the risk of compartment syndrome in this type of injury? Does this alter the indication for regional anesthesia?

Approximately 10% of calcaneal fractures develop compartment syndromes of the foot, particularly those with compression injuries. While relatively rare, this can lead to deformity and neurovascular dysfunction. Diagnosis is often made clinically on the basis of increasing firmness and pain in the foot; this can be complicated if there are associated remote injuries, or if pain is being treated with opioids which may blunt the sensorium. Many clinicians have argued that compartment syndrome should not be diagnosed clinically, but rather by invasive catheterization of compartments at risk. The use of regional anesthetic blocks in this population is controversial: many surgeons and anesthesiologists believe that a sensory block may mask a developing compartment syndrome by preventing the perception of pain. The literature to date does not support this view. In fact, there are multiple reports of regional anesthesia facilitating the diagnosis of compartment syndrome with the onset of pain that has broken through the previously established analgesia (see full discussion in Chapter 6).

What nerves should be blocked to provide adequate sensory block for ankle surgery?

Surgery at the ankle requires blockade of both the tibial and common peroneal nerves, which is usually accomplished by performing a single sciatic block. This can be performed at any point along its course, from parasacral to subgluteal to popliteal fossa, and covers the entire leg below the knee with the exception of a medial strip of skin that extends approximately to the medial malleolus. This is supplied by the saphenous nerve and, if incisions are to be made on the medial side of the ankle, a supplementary saphenous nerve block is performed. The vertebral fracture warrants spinal precautions, and positioning should be managed

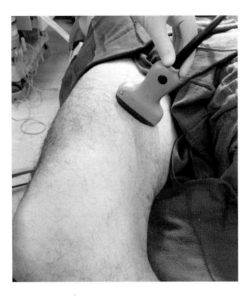

Figure 17.1 Transducer position for ultrasound-guided anterior sciatic nerve block.

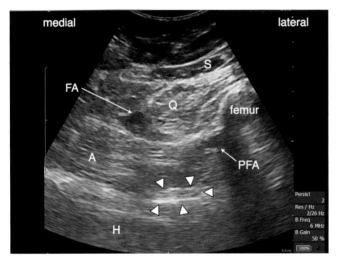

Figure 17.2 Sonoanatomy relevant to the anterior sciatic nerve block. The nerve (arrowheads) is visualized readily in the plane between the adductor muscle group (A) and the hamstrings (H). FA, Femoral artery; PFA, profunda femoris artery; Q, quadriceps muscle group; S, sartorius muscle.

with care. Rolling of the patient is associated with risk of further spinal injury, and these blocks may best be performed in the supine position. The sciatic nerve can be readily blocked in the supine position by using a lateral approach at the popliteal fossa or an anterior approach at mid-femur (Figures 17.1 and 17.2). There are multiple approaches to the saphenous nerve, including subcutaneous infiltration below the tibial plateau or above the medial malleolus, or via a subsartorial approach in the distal thigh (please refer to Chapter 20).

What are the implications of the L2 burst fracture for your anesthetic management?

Burst fractures are relatively common (17% of all spinal fractures) and usually involve retropulsion of osseous fragments into the spinal canal. However, approximately 70% of patients with burst fractures have a normal neurologic exam. In these cases, the decision to pursue operative versus conservative management such as casting or bracing is controversial, and is based on factors such as degree of kyphotic deformity, severity of canal impingement or the presence of posterior column involvement.

Ideally, a thorough sensorimotor neurologic exam is performed by the anesthesiologist prior to induction and any deficits documented. In contrast to a lateral disk herniation, burst fractures typically compress the central canal rather than nerve roots, and so deficits of any spinal level distal to L1 could be present. In this case, since there is no radiographic evidence of canal compromise and the clinical exam is normal, the likelihood of neurologic deterioration is extremely low. Particular attention should be paid to the distribution of any planned nerve blocks. A screening neurologic exam of the peroneal nerve (dorsiflexion, sensory testing of the lateral leg) and tibial nerve (plantar flexion, sensory testing of sole of foot/toes) in this case is indicated.

The patient requests sciatic nerve blocks for pain control. He asks that these be done before he awakens from general anesthesia.

What are the risks and benefits of complying with this request?

Blocks in anesthetized patients have traditionally been discouraged, based on the notion that awake patients are able to report paresthesias, which may signify needle–nerve contact and/ or intraneural injection. Many anesthesiologists feel that, since an anesthetized patient is unable to provide sensory feedback, the potential risk of nerve injury outweighs any benefits conferred by the block. This was highlighted by a series of four cases reported by Benumof (2000) of interscalene brachial plexus blocks performed under general anesthesia that resulted in spinal cord injury and permanent neurologic disability. Some anesthesiologists also contend that a conscious patient may serve as an "early warning system" for the premonitory signs of local anesthetic systemic toxicity (dizziness, tinnitus, circumoral numbness, etc.) and, that by masking these symptoms with heavy sedation or general anesthesia, the patient may be placed at higher risk for serious cardiovascular effects.

On the other hand, anesthetized patients are immobile, which may provide a level of safety compared to a patient who can react to stimuli and move unexpectedly; this is why blocks are typically performed in anesthetized rather than conscious children. In the trauma setting, where 50% of patients are intoxicated, immobility is a potential advantage when nerve blocks are indicated in the uncooperative patient.

Patient comfort is another potential benefit of performing blocks in anesthetized patients. While many nerve blocks are superficial procedures with little associated pain, deep blocks such as sciatic or infraclavicular, or those requiring 18–19-gauge catheter needles can be uncomfortable. The analgesia required to make the traumatically injured patient comfortable for an "awake" block procedure may lead to respiratory embarrassment; many times it is prudent to induce general anesthesia and secure the airway prior to administering opioids and other sedative drugs.

There is some recent evidence that general anesthesia may be protective against local anesthetic-induced cardiotoxicity compared to the awake state. Copeland and colleagues (2008) administered various local anesthetic infusions to conscious and anesthetized sheep, and found that all anesthetized animals survived doses that were lethal in 15–27% of conscious sheep. The mechanism for this is unclear, but may be related to the decreased sympathetic response under general anesthesia, resulting in reduced myocardial irritability.

What is the evidence to support the view that paresthesias reliably predict nerve injury?

While there are several case reports of nerve injury associated with block-related paresthesia, the literature to date shows that the paresthesia during the performance of peripheral nerve blocks is neither sensitive nor specific in predicting subsequent neural injury (Table 17.1). There is no clear relationship between the patient's subjective experience of a paresthesia and subsequent nerve injury – many nerve injuries occur in the absence of paresthesias, while the majority of paresthesias are not associated with nerve damage.

Are there other problems with relying on a patient's report of paresthesia as a monitor of possible intraneural injection?

One of the principal problems with relying on a neurologic response to warn against injury is that, by the time a pain or paresthesia response is elicited, the damage may have been done.

Table 17.1 Investigations with data relating to paresthesia and nerve injury

Study	n	Design	Findings
Bigeleisen (2006)	26	Prospectively placed needles within nerves at the axilla under ultrasound guidance and attempted intraneural injection with 2–3 ml of local anesthetic	Performed 72 intraneural injections, 66 of which had associated paresthesias. No neurologic sequelae immediately postoperatively or at 6 months
Bigeleisen et al. (2009)	39	Prospective study of stimulating current required at both an extraneural and intraneural needletip position during supraclavicular block	All patients received a 5-ml intraneural injection. Two patients experienced pain on injection (5%), but both had normal neurologic exam during postoperative evaluation
Fanelli et al. (1999)	3996	Prospective study of failure rate and complications in axillary, interscalene and sciatic/femoral blocks	Overall rate of neurologic dysfunction 1.7%; rate not influenced by presence or absence of paresthesia during block placement
Robards et al. (2009)	24	Prospective study of relationship between stimulating current and needle to nerve distance. Needletip location recorded with ultrasound	All patients experienced puncture of the sciatic nerve and intraneural injection. Paresthesias were reported in two patients (8%). No neurologic dysfuction following resolution of the block
Sala-Blanch et al. (2011)	17	Prospective study of clinical and electrophysiologic injury following sciatic nerve block	Post-block analysis of ultrasound and CT imaging determined that 16 of 17 patients (94%) received an intraneural injection. There were no paresthesias in any patient, and all patients had normal block recovery

Table 17.2 Objective monitors to prevent nerve injury

Monitor	Contribution	Reference
Electrical nerve stimulation	If motor response at <0.2 mA, can assume needle is intraneural; however, may be intraneural and have *no* motor response (*i.e. highly specific, but insensitive*)	Chan *et al.* (2007) Tsai *et al.* (2008)
Ultrasonography	Can visualize injectate in correct tissue plane (i.e. may rule out intravascular, intraneural). However, even when used by a skilled operator, correct location of the needletip can be misinterpreted	Neal (2010)
Injection pressure monitoring	If low resistance to injection (<20 psi or 1034 mmHg), can assume needle is *not* located inside fascicle; however, high injection pressure may be due to needletip against bone, fascia, plugging of shaft, etc. (*i.e. high sensitivity but non-specific*)	Hadzic *et al.* (2004) Tsui *et al.* (2008)

It has been shown that as little as a fraction of a milliliter injected intraneurally is all that is required to cause permanent nerve injury in animal models. Data from closed claims analysis shows that in many cases where an injection caused pain and was halted immediately, injury still occurred.

Pain and/or paresthesia are often difficult to assess; as pain thresholds vary amongst patients, confusion exists as to what constitutes injurious pain versus so-called "pressure paresthesia." This is especially true of the trauma population, who may have a depressed level of consciousness from sedatives and analgesics administered in the field and in the emergency department.

What other monitors are available to prevent nerve injury during nerve blockade in anesthetized patients?

Instead of relying on subjective symptoms to determine the needle/nerve relationship, there are several objective monitors that can aid in reducing the risk of neural injury during peripheral nerve block. Each one provides different information and hence are complementary. These are outlined in Table 17.2.

References and further reading

Bajammal, S., Tornetta, P., 3rd, Sanders, D., Bhandari, M. (2005). Displaced intra-articular calcaneal fractures. *Journal of Orthopaedic Trauma*, **19**, 360–4.

Benumof, J. L. (2000). Permanent loss of cervical spinal cord function associated with interscalene block performed under general anesthesia. *Anesthesiology*, **93**, 1541–4.

Bigeleisen, P. E. (2006). Nerve puncture and apparent intraneural injection during ultrasound-guided axillary block does not invariably result in neurologic injury. *Anesthesiology*, **105**, 779–83.

Bigeleisen, P. E., Moayeri, N., Groen, G. J. (2009). Extraneural versus intraneural stimulation thresholds during ultrasound-guided supraclavicular block. *Anesthesiology*, **110**, 1235–43.

Chan, V. W. S., Brull, R., McCartney, C. J. L. *et al.* (2007). An ultrasonographic and histological study of intraneural injection and electrical stimulation in pigs. *Anesthesia and Analgesia*, **104**, 1281–4, tables of contents.

Copeland, S. E., Ladd, L. A., Gu, X.-Q., Mather, L. E. (2008). The effects of general anesthesia on the central nervous and cardiovascular system toxicity of local anesthetics. *Anesthesia and Analgesia*, **106**, 1429–39, table of contents.

Fanelli, G., Casati, A., Garancini, P., Torri, G. (1999). Nerve stimulator and multiple injection technique for upper and lower limb blockade: failure rate, patient acceptance, and neurologic complications. Study Group on Regional Anesthesia. *Anesthesia and Analgesia*, **88**, 847–52.

Hadzic, A., Dilberovic, F., Shah, S. *et al.* (2004). Combination of intraneural injection and high injection pressure leads to fascicular injury and neurologic deficits in dogs. *Regional Anesthesia and Pain Medicine*, **29**, 417–23.

Neal, J. M. (2010). Ultrasound-guided regional anesthesia and patient safety: An evidence-based analysis. *Regional Anesthesia and Pain Medicine*, **35**, S59–67.

Rajasekaran, S. (2010). Thoracolumbar burst fractures without neurological deficit: the role for conservative treatment. *European Spine Journal: Official Publication of the European Spine Society, the European Spinal Deformity Society, and the European Section of the Cervical Spine Research Society*, **19**, S40–7.

Robards, C., Hadzic, A., Somasundaram, L., *et al.* (2009). Intraneural injection with low-current stimulation during popliteal sciatic nerve block. *Anesthesia and Analgesia*, **109**, 673–7.

Sala-Blanch, X., Lopez, A. M., Pomes, J. *et al.* (2011) No clinical or electrophysiologic evidence of nerve injury after intraneural injection during sciatic popliteal block. *Anesthesiology*, **115**, 589–95.

Tsai, T. P., Vuckovic, I., Dilberovic, F. *et al.* (2008). Intensity of the stimulating current may not be a reliable indicator of intraneural needle placement. *Regional Anesthesia and Pain Medicine*, **33**, 207–10.

Tsui, B. C. H., Knezevich, M. P., Pillay, J. J. (2008). Reduced injection pressures using a compressed air injection technique (CAIT): an in vitro study. *Regional Anesthesia and Pain Medicine*, **33**, 168–73.

Regional anesthesia and traumatic limb amputation

Key aspects of case

1. Damage control resuscitation.
2. Acute versus chronic stump and phantom limb pain.

Case presentation

A 55-year-old homeless male is brought to the regional trauma center after falling from a slow-moving train. He arrives intubated and with a GCS of 6, with the following vitals: HR 101, BP 82/48, RR 14, T 35.4°C, SpO$_2$ 97% on 100% O$_2$. His injuries include three broken ribs on the left side, a left-sided simple pneumothorax, an open fracture of his left radius and a complete amputation of his left leg approximately 10 cm below the knee joint. There is a tourniquet on his left thigh applied by the paramedics. Pupils are equal but sluggish. He is resuscitated with crystalloid and type-specific packed cells, a chest drain is placed and other life-threatening injuries are ruled out. Once stabilized, the patient is transferred urgently to the operating room for irrigation, debridement and control of hemorrhage related to the amputation.

Case discussion

What are the initial resuscitation goals for this patient?

For decades, aggressive fluid resuscitation with crystalloid followed by packed red blood cells (pRBCs) to maintain a normal arterial blood pressure was the traditional model for ensuring adequate perfusion to vital organs in the exsanguinating patient. However, multiple studies of traumatic hemorrhage in both animals and humans have shown that this strategy leads to increased blood loss, decreased survival and a greater incidence of postoperative complications. The reason that early large volume resuscitation leads to poorer outcomes likely relates to decreased blood viscosity, dilution of coagulation factors and hydrostatic disruption of any clot that initially formed after the initial injury. Modern thinking in non-surgical trauma care focuses on treating all three arms of the "lethal triad" of hypothermia, acidosis and coagulopathy in what is termed "damage control resuscitation." This is so-named to emphasize its pairing with damage control surgical techniques, and consists of the following.

- **Permissive hypotension:** injured blood vessels rely on a combination of the coagulation cascade, hypotension and vessel spasm to stop hemorrhage. For example, a well-known phenomenon is for traumatic limb amputations to arrive at hospital with minimal bleeding, only to bleed extensively once arterial pressure has been corrected to normal levels with aggressive fluid infusion. In damage control resuscitation, systolic pressures are kept at 80–90 mmHg until bleeding can be surgically controlled.

2. **Normothermia:** the deleterious effects of hypothermia on the coagulation cascade (leading to ↑bleeding, worsening of acidosis, etc.) have been well described. A team approach to preventing hypothermia is the rule in most trauma systems now, starting from passive insulation in the prehospital setting to heated trauma bays and operating rooms, to aggressive fluid warming and forced air warmers.

3. **Acidosis:** patients in hemorrhagic shock are frequently acidotic, which has been shown to directly reduce fibrinogen concentration, platelet counts, and activated factor X and thrombin generation. Strategies are aimed less at correcting acidosis with agents such as bicarbonate or tromethamine (THAM) (both of which have mixed results), and more at preventing worsening acid–base status. Examples include preventing hypercarbia and the avoidance of normal saline as a resuscitation fluid.

4. **Blood product ratios:** recent studies have shown that the traditional emphasis on crystalloid as a resuscitation fluid followed by pRBCs at a certain threshold leads to delayed resolution of the coagulopathy and an increased need for blood products. Instead, a central tenet of damage control resuscitation is the early use of plasma and pRBCs in a 1:1, or similar, ratio.

It is important to note that damage control resuscitation is intended for penetrating trauma or the exsanguinating injured patient. There is no evidence supporting its use in blunt trauma, and permissive hypotension may be hazardous in head-injured or pregnant patients.

Is there a specific role for regional anesthesia/analgesia in traumatic amputation?

Amputation is associated with severe acute pain that can develop into one or more of three long-term phenomena.

1. **Stump pain:** this is localized to the site of amputation and can be either acute (nociceptive) or chronic (neuropathic).

2. **Phantom sensation:** defined as the sensory perception of a missing body part without pain.

3. **Phantom limb pain:** defined as a noxious sensory phenomenon in the missing limb. It is thought to occur in 30–85% of patients after limb amputation and usually occurs in the distal limb.

There is a strong role for continuous regional anesthetic techniques (epidural or peripheral nerve catheter) for treatment of acute postoperative pain. What is less clear is the effectiveness of regional anesthetic techniques on reducing chronic stump or phantom limb pain. The results of a recent systematic review suggest that pre-emptive analgesia of any type has little effect on chronic pain after amputation. However, individual studies have reported more encouraging results. Gehling and Tryba (2003) showed that perioperative epidural analgesia reduced the incidence of severe phantom limb pain. In a retrospective study of 64 patients, Grant and Wood (2008) demonstrated a decrease in phantom limb pain incidence after amputation in those patients receiving continuou sciatic nerve blocks. Recently, Karanikolas *et al.* (2011) found that 48 hours of effective analgesia (epidural *or* IV opioids) prior to *and* after amputation resulted in a significantly reduced incidence and severity of phantom limb pain. Finally, Borghi and colleagues (2010) performed an observational study of amputation patients who received continuous sciatic blockade for a mean of 30 days, and reported a reduction in severe phantom limb pain to zero in 97% of patients.

What are the implications of the transected nerves in the development of chronic pain?

Neuromas are disorganized proliferations of nerve fascicles, and are an inevitable outcome of the complete transection of a peripheral nerve during traumatic amputation, especially if located near the stump. Symptomatic neuromas are a common indication for amputation revision, and can be exquisitely painful – even normal physiologic stimuli such as stretching or pressure can be experienced as moderate to severe pain. This limits the effectiveness of a prosthesis, and results in an impaired quality of life.

At the time of completion of the amputation, the nerves should undergo traction neurectomy so that the new severed nerve stump retracts well away from the weightbearing portion of the terminal residual limb. Despite this, some neuromas still cause chronic pain. Ultrasound-guided neuroma blocks have been used successfully to treat this phenomenon.

You decide to perform combined sciatic and femoral catheters for this patient at the end of the case while still under general anesthesia.

Which approach is best in this circumstance for the sciatic catheter?

There are three common approaches for sciatic catheters: subgluteal, popliteal and anterior. This last approach is rarely used in our practice because the distance from the anterior surface of the thigh to the nerve is not insignificant, and the degree of muscle trauma with a large-bore needle is that much greater. This is especially relevant in the setting of coagulopathy. Other considerations that factor into sciatic approach include:

- **The type of amputation:** both approaches (popliteal and subgluteal) are suitable for amputations below the knee, although if the popliteal approach is chosen, the free end of the catheter should be secured away from the surgical field. There will be some longitudinal movement of the nerve if traction neurectomy is performed, but this is only a theoretical factor, and our experience is that popliteal catheters remain in good location afterwards. Above the knee amputations should obviously receive a more proximal approach.

- **Spinal precautions:** if there is a potential for spinal injury, logrolling the patient is an unnecessary hazard that should be minimized. Popliteal block should be chosen if possible.

- **Patient size:** the size and shape of the leg sometimes dictates the best approach. In the obese, the popliteal is usually the easiest approach of the three.

The lateral thigh just above the popliteal crease is abraded and lacerated. You decide to perform a subgluteal catheter instead.

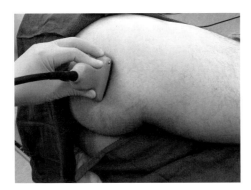

Figure 18.1 Transducer position for ultrasound-guided subgluteal sciatic nerve block.

What are the technical considerations for performing an ultrasound-guided continuous subgluteal sciatic nerve block?

- Positioning is often an issue, as this block is best performed in the lateral decubitus position with the hip and knee somewhat flexed to allow access to the upper thigh and buttock. Inability to perform this maneuver for whatever reason should prompt the consideration of an alternative approach.

- If nerve stimulation is to be used at the same time, exposure of the calf and foot are required to observe motor responses – this is not an option in this case, but a hamstring motor response is often sufficient.

- After skin disinfection, the round, bony prominences of the greater trochanter and ischial tuberosity are palpated, and a curvilinear transducer placed in a transverse orientation in the depression between the two bones (Figure 18.1).

- The sciatic nerve is visualized in its short axis between the two hyperechoic bony prominences. The gluteus maximus muscle is seen as the most superficial muscular layer bridging the two bones, and is usually several centimeters thick. The sciatic nerve is located immediately deep to the gluteus maximus, superficial to the quadratus femoris muscle. At this location in the thigh, it is seen as an oval or roughly triangular, hyperechoic structure (Figure 18.2).

- If the nerve is not immediately apparent, tilting the transducer proximally or distally can often help to improve the contrast and bring the nerve "out" of the background of the musculature. Alternatively, sliding the transducer slightly proximally or distally may improve the quality of the image.

- Once identified, a 17-GA 10-cm Tuohy needle is inserted in-plane from the lateral aspect of the transducer and advanced towards the sciatic nerve. If nerve stimulation is used, the passage of the needle through the posterior fascial plane of the gluteus maximus is often associated with a motor response of the hamstring muscles, or those of the calf or foot.

- Once the needletip is adjacent to the nerve, a small (5–7-ml) bolus of local anesthetic (LA) is administered to "open up" the space and confirm correct placement. The transducer

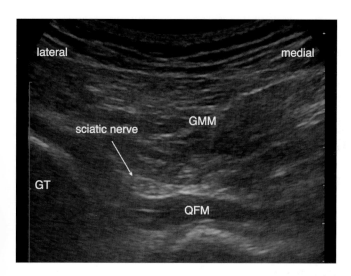

lateral

medial

GMM

sciatic nerve

GT

QFM

Figure 18.2 Sonoanatomy relevant to the subgluteal sciatic nerve block. The nerve is visualized readily in the plane between the gluteus maximus muscle (GMM) and the quadratus femoris muscle (QFM). The principal bony landmark is the greater trochanter (GT) lateral to the nerve.

can then be set aside briefly while the catheter is advanced 1–2 cm beyond the tip of the needle (it is important to know in advance which markings on the catheter equate with catheter emergence through the needletip as it is advanced).

- The needle is removed, and the sciatic nerve imaged again with the transducer. Often the catheter cannot be visualized, but its position can be inferred by bolusing LA and observing the spread next to the nerve. The color Doppler function is also useful for this. Frequently the catheter must be withdrawn a few centimeters if it has been advanced too far.

- The catheter is secured to the skin and connected to an infusion pump programmed to infuse at 10 ml/h. Once the patient can respond to instructions, the programmed rate can change to 5 ml/h with a patient-controlled bolus of 5 ml every 30–45 minutes.

References and further reading

Beekley, A. C. (2008). Damage control resuscitation: a sensible approach to the exsanguinating surgical patient. *Critical Care Medicine*, **36**, S267–74.

Borghi, B., D'Addabbo, M., White, P. F. *et al.* (2010). The use of prolonged peripheral neural blockade after lower extremity amputation: the effect on symptoms associated with phantom limb syndrome. *Anesthesia and Analgesia*, **111**, 1308–15.

Fischler, A. H., Gross, J. B. (2007). Ultrasound-guided sciatic neuroma block for treatment of intractable stump pain. *Journal of Clinical Anesthesia*, **19**, 626–8.

Gehling, M., Tryba, M. (2003). [Prophylaxis of phantom pain: is regional analgesia ineffective?]. *Schmerz*, **17**, 11–19.

Grant, A. J., Wood, C. (2008). The effect of intra-neural local anaesthetic infusion on pain following major lower limb amputation. *Scottish Medical Journal*, **53**, 4–6.

Karanikolas, M., Aretha, D., Tsolakis, I., *et al.* (2011). Optimized perioperative analgesia reduces chronic phantom limb pain intensity, prevalence, and frequency: a prospective, randomized, clinical trial. *Anesthesiology*, **114**, 1144–54.

Tintle, S. M., Keeling, J. J., Shawen, S. B., Forsberg, J. A., Potter, B. K. (2010). Traumatic and trauma-related amputations: part I: general principles and lower-extremity amputations. *The Journal of Bone and Joint Surgery. American Volume*, **92**, 2852–68.

Ypsilantis, E., Tang, T. Y. (2010). Pre-emptive analgesia for chronic limb pain after amputation for peripheral vascular disease: a systematic review. *Annals of Vascular Surgery*, **24**, 1139–46.

Chapter 19

Complications of brachial plexus blockade

Key aspects of case

1. Choice of brachial plexus block approach to minimize pleural puncture.
2. Management of post-block neuropathy.

Case presentation

A 48-year-old woman is brought to the regional trauma center after falling 30 feet (10 m) down a mountainside while hiking. She is awake and responsive, with a GCS of 14, and is maintaining her airway in a semi-rigid collar. She is found to have a right proximal humeral fracture, three broken ribs on the left side and a left-sided hemopneumothorax, for which a chest drain is placed. There are no other significant injuries. After resuscitation and stabilization, she is admitted to hospital and scheduled for an open reduction internal fixation (ORIF) of the humeral fracture the following day. Prior to leaving the trauma bay, you decide to perform ultrasound-guided intercostal blocks to relieve the patient's chest wall pain (please see Chapter 7). Thirty-six hours later the patient arrives at the operating room. Her chest wall pain is well controlled, although her right arm and shoulder are quite painful when she moves. The chest tube is on suction, and the underwater seal is bubbling vigorously with expiration.

Case discussion

What is the implication of the bubbling chest drain?

This patient has a large air leak through the underwater seal, indicating that a communication exists between the tracheobronchial–alveolar tree and the pleural space. In the setting of blunt chest trauma, an air leak should always raise the possibility of a tracheobronchial disruption and resultant bronchopleural fistula. Alternatively, this may simply be an alveolar–pleural communication that will heal on its own and resolve. Differentiation of these two entities is important as the treatment of tracheobronchial rupture is prompt surgical repair versus conservative management for simple alveolar pneumothorax. Flexible fiberoptic bronchoscopy is indicated to make the diagnosis, which in this case showed an intact tracheobronchial tree.

What are the advantages and disadvantages of general anesthesia versus brachial plexus block for this procedure?

In the event of an ongoing air leak, positive pressure ventilation should be avoided if possible to prevent further injury of the small alveolar tear, as well as wasted ventilation. Tension pneumothorax would also be a concern if a chest tube was not in place (e.g. a small pneumothorax being treated conservatively). General anesthesia with spontaneous ventilation is an option, particularly if an extraglottic airway device can be used. There may be patient factors such as a full stomach that preclude this plan. Postoperative pain control following humeral fracture repair under general anesthesia usually requires intravenous opioids, which may impair an already tenuous respiratory state.

Brachial plexus block provides excellent postoperative analgesia, especially if a catheter technique is used. A well-done block plus mild sedation obviates the need to manage the airway. Brachial plexus block has been shown to reduce the incidence of nausea and vomiting, time to ambulation, pain scores and time to discharge readiness in elective upper extremity orthopedic surgery. Phrenic nerve block is a consideration, depending on the approach; interscalene brachial plexus block is associated with a 50–100% rate of phrenic nerve block, depending on the volume of local anesthetic used, whereas the axillary approach is effectively zero. The phrenic nerve block rates for supraclavicular and infraclavicular approaches vary in reports but are between 0% and 60%.

Would a brachial plexus block put the patient at risk for bilateral pneumothoraces?

The risk of pneumothorax is important in this case. The patient already has a contralateral pneumothorax and a second, iatrogenic, pleural puncture may cause her to suffer serious respiratory compromise. The actual risk for brachial plexus block is largely unknown, particularly because the clinical presentation is usually delayed by 10–12 h, and may be subtle. Presumably there are undetected and unreported pneumothoraces that complicate brachial plexus blockade.

The supraclavicular approach has been associated with an incidence of pneumothorax of 0.6–6.1%, although these data are more than 50 years old, included a small number of patients and reflect the rarely used Kulenkampff technique. Two recent prospective case series that include over 3000 patients reported no pneumothoraces with the use of the subclavian perivascular technique. Less is known about the true incidence of this complication via the interscalene and infraclavicular approaches, although both have been reported. Ultrasound guidance has been advocated as a means to reduce this complication further, although it is by no means a guarantee of extrapleural needle placement; pneumothoraces have been described with both ultrasound-guided supraclavicular and infraclavicular blocks.

Particularly in this case, where a contralateral pneumothorax already exists, it seems prudent to avoid the approach that brings the needletip closest to the pleura. Of the four common approaches, the supraclavicular and infraclavicular both require deposition of local anesthetic in close proximity to the chest wall (Figure 19.1), whereas interscalene and axillary enjoy a larger anatomical margin of safety for pneumothorax.

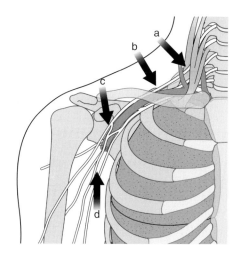

Figure 19.1 Coronal section of the chest showing the relationship of different approaches to the brachial plexus and the proximity to the chest wall. Anatomically, the interscalene (a) and axillary (d) approaches are less likely to result in pneumothorax than the supraclavicular (b) and infraclavicular (c) approaches.

What are the practical considerations for performance of brachial plexus block in patients with a proximal humeral fracture?

This is a painful fracture and mobilization of the limb should be minimized if possible. For this reason, axillary brachial plexus block is not ideal, as it requires abduction of the arm. Likewise, if nerve stimulation is used, a low (e.g. <0.5 mA) current intensity should be set prior to inserting the needle so that the motor response is not excessive. In our institution, we frequently keep the stimulator turned off during needle advancement under ultrasound, and only turn it on for confirmation once the needle is "parked" next to the nerve. Patient positioning and ergonomics are important and, if possible, the patient should be placed in the most comfortable position that permits adequate access to the needle insertion site. The semilateral position is often a good compromise of these two goals.

You perform an uneventful single injection interscalene block. Two days later you are called to see the patient because she is complaining of residual numbness along the lateral aspect of the volar arm and forearm. Examination reveals normal power in the right arm but paresthesia in the C5/C6 distribution.

What is your course of action?

Nerve injury is a feared complication of regional anesthesia. There are several key mechanisms of injury related to nerve blocks, including mechanical trauma from the needle, direct toxicity from local anesthetics (especially if injected intraneurally) and ischemia from vasoconstrictors such as epinephrine. However, neurologic dysfunction following peripheral nerve block is not always a result of the anesthetic and may be related to vascular injury, compression from tourniquets or casts, or an injury related to positioning or surgical trauma. Pre-existing subclinical neuropathy may also play a role in the development of symptoms after surgery (e.g. double-crush syndrome). Once a clinician has been alerted to the deficit, meticulous follow-up care and attention to the patient's symptoms and concerns goes a long way towards a positive resolution of the problem.

The vast majority of "prolonged blocks" and mild sensory neuropathies resolve spontaneously with time, usually disappearing within 2–6 weeks, although a small fraction require

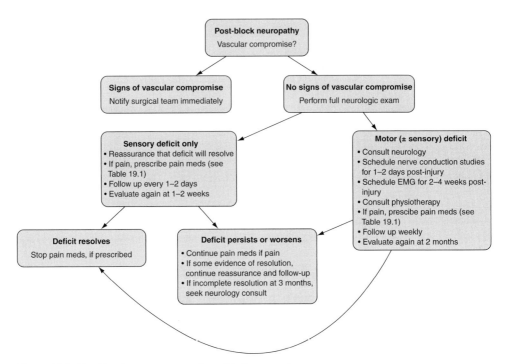

Figure 19.2 Algorithm for management of post-block neuropathy.

up to 3 months or more to resolve completely. A motor deficit is an indication to consult neurology, as this represents a more serious prognosis. An algorithm for the management of post-block neuropathies is outlined in Figure 19.2. Note that vascular injury must be ruled out first, as this is a reversible cause that can have devastating consequences if not corrected immediately.

Neurologic studies are indicated if a patient has a motor deficit or if a sensory deficit fails to resolve. There are two types of electrophysiologic tests that can help delineate the nature of a nerve lesion, particularly where it is and how long it has been present.

1. **Nerve conduction studies:** these are performed by stimulating cutaneous electrodes and recording the neural activity downstream along the course of a nerve. The conduction velocity between the two points is calculated and the amplitude of the response measured. A reduction in conduction velocity indicates myelin damage, whereas a decrease in amplitude suggests axonal damage. A nerve lesion can be detected as soon as 1–2 days after the injury, which is when these studies should be performed. If abnormal, the lesion should be localized using electromyography.

2. **Electromyography (EMG):** this test is performed by recording myoelectrical activity from small electrodes placed in target muscles. For example, if the musculocutaneous nerve has shown abnormalities on nerve conduction studies, an EMG of the biceps brachii should be performed. However, the lesion may be more proximal (i.e. at the level of the superior trunk) and so testing several other muscles (e.g. deltoid, pectoralis) is suggested to confirm the location of the injury. Normally innervated muscles show no

Table 19.1 Medications commonly prescribed for management of neuropathic pain

Medication	Clinical notes
	First-line treatment
Tricyclic antidepressants	• E.g. amitriptyline, nortriptyline, imipramine, desipramine • Multiple actions: blocks reuptake of serotonin, norepinephrine, NMDA receptors and sodium channels • Side effects: dry mouth, constipation, blurred vision, orthostasis, sedation, QT interval prolongation
Serotonin–norepinephrine reuptake inhibitors (SNRIs)	• E.g. venlafaxine, duloxetine • Side effects: drowsiness, dizziness, fatigue, headache, blurred vision, urinary retention
Gabapentin/pregabalin	• Blocks neuronal calcium channels, altering balance of inhibitory and excitatory pathways • Side effects: drowsiness, sedation
	Second-line treatment
Tramadol	• Mu agonist activity; also norepinephrine and serotonin reuptake inhibition • Low incidence of constipation compared with other opioids • Minimal risk of abuse
Opioids	• Oxycodone most commonly studied and prescribed • High abuse potential
Capsaicin ointment	• Vanilloid compound found in hot peppers • Burns when initially applied, limiting patient acceptance

spontaneous activity on EMG; after 2–4 weeks of denervation, spontaneous fibrillation will occur. Some clinicians suggest that EMG testing be done in the first few days after an injury to rule out pre-existing neuromuscular injury, as a new lesion will take several weeks to manifest.

If the patient complains of pain as part of their syndrome, he/she should be offered medications that treat neuropathic pain (Table 19.1). This is usually best done by referral to a chronic pain specialist or neurologist.

Further reading

Aminoff, M. J. (2004). Electrophysiologic testing for the diagnosis of peripheral nerve injuries. *Anesthesiology*, **100**, 1298–303.

Attal, N., Cruccu, G., Baron, R. *et al.* (2010). EFNS guidelines on the pharmacological treatment of neuropathic pain: 2010 revision. *European Journal of Neurology: The Official Journal of the European Federation of Neurological Societies*, **17**, 1113–e88.

Bhatia, A., Lai, J., Chan, V. W. S., Brull, R. (2010). Case report: pneumothorax as a complication of the ultrasound-guided supraclavicular approach for brachial plexus block. *Anesthesia and Analgesia*, **111**, 817–19.

Borgeat, A., Aguirre, J., Curt, A. (2010). Case scenario: neurologic complication after continuous interscalene block. *Anesthesiology*, **112**, 742–5.

Crews, J. C., Gerancher, J. C., Weller, R. S. (2007). Pneumothorax after coracoid infraclavicular brachial plexus block. *Anesthesia and Analgesia*, **105**, 275–7.

Neal, J. M. (2010). Ultrasound-guided regional anesthesia and patient safety: An evidence-based analysis. *Regional Anesthesia and Pain Medicine*, **35**, S59–S67.

Sanchez, H. B., Mariano, E. R., Abrams, R., Meunier, M. (2008). Pneumothorax following infraclavicular brachial plexus block for hand surgery. *Orthopedics*, **31**, 709.

Sugiura, T., Akiyoshi, R., Kato, R., Sasano, H., Sobue, K. (2011). [Interscalene block combined with general anesthesia under spontaneous breathing in a patient with a giant bulla]. *Masui. The Japanese Journal of Anesthesiology*, **60**, 1101–3.

Chapter 20

Regional anesthesia and trauma in pregnancy

Key aspects of case

1. Management of trauma in the pregnant patient.
2. Regional techniques for distal tibia fracture.

Case presentation

A 24-year-old pregnant woman who is G1P0 at 36 weeks' gestation falls at home while descending a staircase. She strikes her head, neck and back before landing on her left ankle. Her husband calls an ambulance, and she is brought to the emergency room where she is extremely anxious and frightened, but able to respond appropriately, with a GCS of 15. She complains of generalized pain all over, but especially in her lower back and left ankle, which has an obvious valgus deformity. Her vital signs are HR 111, BP 146/89, RR 20, T 37.0C. The fetal monitor shows a fetal heart rate of 145 with appropriate variability. FAST scan shows no free fluid in the abdomen, her pelvis appears stable and there is no bleeding or amniotic fluid from the vagina. Lab work reveals a hemoglobin of 10.5 mg/dl; the remainder of the bloodwork was within normal limits. An MRI of her spine shows no bony or soft-tissue injury. Plain films of her left ankle show a bimalleolar fracture.

Case discussion

What is the epidemiology of trauma in pregnancy?

Trauma is the most common cause of maternal death during pregnancy in the developed world. Since most injuries are minor and unreported, the actual incidence is unknown, but data from trauma registries suggests that it occurs in 6–7% of all pregnancies. Motor vehicle accidents are still the leading cause of trauma in this group, although domestic violence is relatively frequent, occurring in up to 30% of all pregnancies. Ignoring injuries related to the gravid uterus, pregnant women are more likely to incur serious abdominal injuries, but less likely to suffer head or chest injuries compared to non-pregnant patients.

What are the considerations regarding the initial management of the pregnant trauma patient?

Pregnancy causes significant physiologic and anatomic changes that influence both the evaluation of the patient, as well as the approach and responses to resuscitation (Table 20.1). Since

Table 20.1 Physiologic and anatomic changes of pregnancy and their impact on initial resuscitation

Physiologic changes (at term)	Significance in trauma
Airway swelling and friability	Difficult mask ventilation, intubation; airway bleeding
Minute ventilation ↑by 45% ($PaCO_2$=30 mmHg)	A "normal" $PaCO_2$ may signify impending respiratory failure
↓ Functional residual capacity by 20%	Prone to rapid desaturation
↑ Blood volume by 45%, relative ↓ in Hb (11–12 g/dl)	May lose 1200–1500 ml of blood before showing signs of hypovolemia
↑ Cardiac output by 50%	May mask hypovolemia
Aortocaval compression by uterus	Need for left uterine displacement during resuscitation
Hypercoagulable state	Prone to thrombosis
Pituitary gland ↑ up to 50% in size	Shock may cause pituitary infarction
Gravid uterus extends up to costal margin	Uterus, fetus and placenta at risk for blunt abdominal trauma; bowel pushed cephalad and more protected by ribs
Fetal head within pelvis (if vertex)	Pelvic fracture may result in skull fracture/intracranial injury
Widening of symphysis pubis and sacroiliac joints	Must take into account when interpreting pelvic films

there are two patients involved, the mother and fetus, fetal monitoring and coordinated multidisciplinary care with anesthesiologists, trauma surgeons, obstetricians and emergency medicine physicians is essential; however, the first priority lies in the resuscitation of the mother, as optimum care of the mother ensures the best chance for the fetus. Continuous fetal monitoring with a cardiotocodynamometer is recommended after 20–24 weeks' gestation.

Initial treatment priorities for an injured pregnant patient are essentially the same as for the non-pregnant patient (i.e. the airway still needs to be evaluated and addressed first). Diagnostic peritoneal lavage is rarely used for evaluation of significant abdominal injury in these patients because of the risk of injuring the uterus, although the open, supraumbilical approach has been used safely. FAST scanning involves no radiation and is non-invasive for this purpose. Sonographic examination of the uterus, placenta and fetus should be performed whenever possible, both to confirm fetal wellbeing and to rule out life-threatening conditions such as placental abruption and uterine rupture. The use of X-rays and CT scanning should not be withheld because of the pregnancy if indicated in the care of the mother, but lead shielding of the abdomen should be undertaken when feasible to reduce the overall exposure. Finally, there are cases during maternal cardiopulmonary arrest in which Cesarean delivery may at least save the life of the fetus. In these situations, the success rate for perimortem Cesarean delivery plummets dramatically after 5 minutes, and prompt intervention with continuing CPR is crucial to a good neonatal outcome.

What is the disposition of pregnant patients following minor trauma?

Many pregnant patients with minor trauma can be discharged home following a period of at least 6 hours of fetal monitoring, especially if the mechanism of injury does not involve the abdomen and pelvis. If the following occur at any time, admission and further care by an obstetrician is warranted:

- Uterine contractions/irritability
- Non-reassuring fetal heart rate pattern
- Vaginal bleeding, amniotic fluid leakage, or abdominal pain or cramping
- Evidence of hypovolemia.

The patient is transferred to the antenatal floor for observation, while awaiting open reduction internal fixation (ORIF) of her ankle fracture scheduled for the following morning. You go to see her in preparation for her surgery and find her very anxious about receiving an anesthetic.

What are the considerations surrounding general anesthesia in the pregnant patient?

Despite concern on the part of physicians and patients regarding the effect of anesthesia on the outcome of pregnancy, no anesthetic drug has been shown to be clearly teratogenic to the fetus. Early studies of nitrous oxide and benzodiazepines suggesting an association with birth defects were found to be either heavily confounded or subsequently refuted. However, it is prudent to expose the fetus to as few agents as possible, especially with recent evidence suggesting accelerated neuronal apoptosis in immature rodent brains, with associated behavioral changes. Also relevant is the small increase in the risk of miscarriage or preterm delivery following non-obstetric surgery in pregnant patients.

Other considerations include the added challenge of a full stomach, decreased functional residual capacity with a tendency to rapid desaturation, a significantly increased risk of difficult or failed airway, and increased minimum alveolar concentration for the volatile anesthetics. The most important priorities during any anesthetic in a pregnant patient are to maintain adequate oxygenation and systemic arterial blood pressure (owing to the relatively passive dependence of the uteroplacental circulation).

You speak with the patient and agree on a peripheral nerve block technique. Which nerves require blocking for ORIF of a bimalleolar fracture?

The sciatic nerve innervates all of the leg below the knee with the exception of a variable cutaneous strip running from the knee down to the area of the medial malleolus – this is innervated by the saphenous nerve, the terminal branch of the femoral nerve. Any procedure involving an incision over the medial malleolus should prompt the blockade of the saphenous nerve (or the femoral nerve, which results in a saphenous nerve block). The ideal combination of blocks for this procedure is a sciatic (at any level) plus a saphenous nerve block.

What influences the choice of approach to the sciatic nerve? Is a saphenous block as good as a femoral block?

The sciatic nerve can be blocked from the parasacral area proximally right down to the popliteal fossa, and any of these approaches provide excellent anesthesia/analagesia to all of the leg below the knee (except the cutaneous territory of the saphenous nerve). The more proximal approaches (such as subgluteal or parasacral) are also likely to block the posterior cutaneous nerve of the thigh, although for most indications cutaneous analgesia of the posterior thigh has little significance. In addition, the more proximal the block, the more motor units of the hamstrings are blocked. While this may have little significance peri-operatively, hamstring impairment can adversely affect patient satisfaction if an extended duration block is planned, as it is more difficult to make minor adjustments in position for comfort postoperatively.

Positioning is important in trauma for reasons of comfort and maintenance of spinal or other skeletal immobility. For this reason, unless contraindicated, we usually favor a supine approach to the sciatic nerve in our institution, via either the popliteal approach or the anterior approach (see Chapter 17).

A similar argument can be made for performing a saphenous nerve block distally; since fewer motor fibers are blocked compared with femoral block, the patient still receives excellent analgesia while retaining the ability to extend the knee, which increases patient satisfaction. One caveat is that some approaches to the saphenous block are associated with poor success rates – for example, the commonly performed approach involving subcutaneous infiltration below the medial condyle of the tibia often leads to disappointing results. A newer approach using ultrasound has been associated with a very high success rate.

You elect to perform a popliteal sciatic block and a subsartorial saphenous nerve block for this procedure using ultrasound guidance for both.

What are the technical considerations in performing these blocks?

- The patient can be positioned in the left semilateral position, which achieves both uterine displacement off the inferior vena cava, as well as adequate access for both blocks. The lower hip and knee should be somewhat flexed (Figure 20.1).
- The anteromedial thigh is prepped widely up to the mid-thigh level.

  Block #1: popliteal sciatic
- A linear transducer is placed on the posterior aspect of the popliteal fossa, at the level of the crease. At a depth of 2–3 cm, the popliteal vessels should be obvious; identification may be made easier with color Doppler. Immediately shallow (and often lateral) to the artery is the tibial nerve. The common peroneal nerve can usually be seen near the lateral edge of the monitor. It is common to require some tilting of the transducer to "bring out" the tibial nerve from the background.
- The transducer is then slid proximally several centimeters (Figure 20.2), while observing the gradual merging of the tibial and peroneal nerves within a common sciatic nerve sheath (Figure 20.3). The point at which these two nerves are just about to join is the ideal place to perform the sciatic block, as it reliably and quickly blocks both branches owing to the increased surface area, and the nerve is still relatively shallow (i.e. visible). As the transducer is moved more proximally in the thigh, the nerve becomes deeper and more difficult to image.
- A 10-cm stimulating needle is inserted in-plane from the medial aspect of the transducer and advanced towards the nerves. The goal is to place the needletip in between the

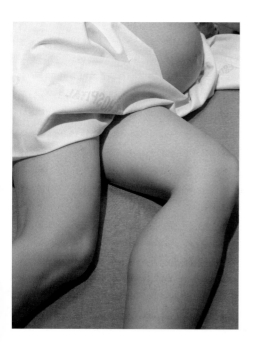

Figure 20.1 One possible positioning solution for popliteal sciatic and saphenous nerve blocks in a pregnant patient. Left lateral tilt exposes the medial thigh which facilitates both blocks and provides uterine displacement from the vena cava.

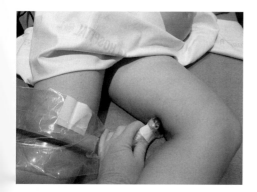

Figure 20.2 Transducer position for ultrasound-guided popliteal sciatic nerve block.

tibial and peroneal nerves and deposit the local anesthetic within the common nerve sheath. If nerve stimulation is used, the contact of the needletip with either nerve is usually associated with a motor response of the calf or foot. After careful aspiration, 1–2 ml of local anesthetic is injected to confirm the proper injection site, followed by the remainder to make up 20 ml in total. A long-acting, high-concentration local anesthetic is indicated for this painful surgical procedure (e.g. ropivacaine 0.5%).

Block #2: subsartorial saphenous
The needle is then removed and the transducer placed on the anteromedial thigh approximately one-third to halfway up the femur (Figure 20.4).

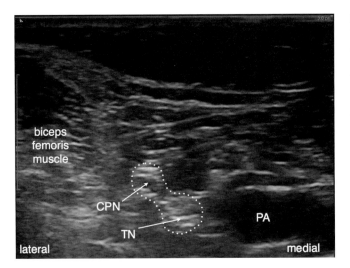

Figure 20.3 Sonoanatomy relevant to the ultrasound-guided popliteal sciatic nerve block. The sciatic nerve is visualized lateral (and slightly superficial) to the popliteal artery (PA). At this level the nerve is just beginning to bifurcate into the tibial (TN) and common peroneal (CPN) portions, but still shares a common sheath.

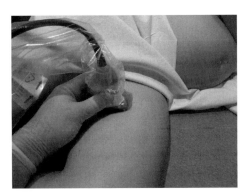

Figure 20.4 Transducer position for ultrasound-guided subsartorial saphenous nerve block. The transducer is placed on the anteromedial thigh, at approximately the mid-femoral level.

- At a similar depth (approximately 3 cm), the femoral artery will be visible sandwiched between the sartorius muscle, the vastus medialis muscle and the adductor longus muscle in the adductor canal (Figure 20.5). The terminal branches of the femoral nerve, namely the saphenous nerve and the motor nerve to the vastus medialis, are also located in the adductor canal. The saphenous nerve is usually on the lateral side of the artery, but travels over the artery to lie on the medial side as they approach the adductor hiatus near the popliteal fossa.
- Once a good view of the femoral artery and adductor canal is obtained, a 10-cm short bevel needle is inserted either out-of-plane or in-plane. One advantage to the out-of-plane approach is that the needle is less likely to injure the vessels when it "pops" through the back wall of the sartorius muscle compared with the in-plane approach if the target is to deposit local anesthetic on the lateral side of the vessel (Figure 20.6).

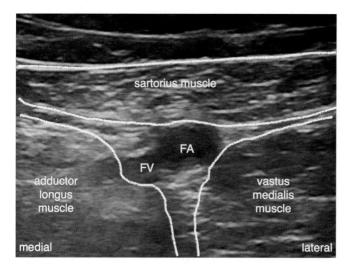

Figure 20.5 Sonoanatomy relevant to the subsartorial saphenous nerve block. The adductor canal is formed by the sartorius muscle superficially, the adductor longus muscle medially and the vastus medialis laterally. In addition to the saphenous nerve (often not visualized), the adductor canal also contains the femoral artery (FA) and vein (FV).

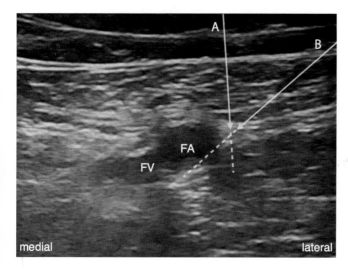

Figure 20.6 Two possible needle paths for the ultrasound-guided subsartorial saphenous nerve block. The out-of-plane approach (A) guards against vascular injury in the case of needle advancement that is inadvertently deep (dashed lines), provided the needle is directed lateral to the artery. Excessive needle depth while using the in-plane approach (B) may result in vascular puncture owing to the projected needle path.

- After aspiration for blood, a small (1–2-ml) bolus of local anesthetic is administered to confirm correct placement, followed by the remainder of a total of 5–10 ml.

Further reading

Chestnut D H, Polley L S, Tsen L C, Wong C A. (2009). *Chestnut's Obstetric Anesthesia: Principles and Practice: Expert Consult - Online and Print*, 4th edn. Philadelphia: Mosby.

Guntz, E., Herman, P., Debizet, E. *et al.* (2004). Sciatic nerve block in the popliteal fossa: description of a new medial approach. *Canadian Journal of Anaesthesia*, **51**, 817–20.

Meroz, Y., Elchalal, U., Ginosar, Y. (2007). Initial trauma management in advanced pregnancy. *Anesthesiology Clinics*, **25**, 117–29.

Mirza, F. G., Devine, P. C., Gaddipati, S. (2010). Trauma in pregnancy: a systematic approach. *American Journal of Perinatology*, **27**, 579–86.

Reitman, E., Flood, P. (2011). Anaesthetic considerations for non-obstetric surgery during pregnancy. *British Journal of Anaesthesia*, **107** Suppl 1, i72–8.

Saranteas, T., Anagnostis, G., Paraskeuopoulos, T. *et al.* (2011). Anatomy and clinical implications of the ultrasound-guided subsartorial saphenous nerve block. *Regional Anesthesia and Pain Medicine*, **36**, 399–402.

Regional anesthesia
and the injured athlete

Key aspects of case

1. Distribution of analgesia with transversus abdominis plane block.
2. Choice of blocks for anterior cruciate ligament repair.

Case presentation

A 19-year-old male elite speed skater is training at an oval course when a collision occurs with another skater, causing both to crash into the boards. Despite wearing a helmet, he suffers a brief loss of consciousness when his head strikes the ice. He is taken to a nearby hospital where he is found to have a GCS of 15, with stable vital signs and no obvious life-threatening injury. Examination reveals a 14-cm laceration of his anterior abdominal wall that extends down to the muscle layer, caused by the other athlete's skate. He also has a swollen and painful left knee. FAST scan and CT of the head and cervical spine are all normal. An attempted exploration of the wound to determine if it extends deep to the peritoneum is unsuccessful owing to continued bleeding and pain. He is taken to the operating room for irrigation, debridement and hemostatic control of his abdominal wound. He is otherwise healthy and last ate a meal 2 hours ago.

Case discussion

What are the anesthetic options for this case?

1. **General anesthesia:** while providing adequate operating conditions for this simple procedure, there are considerations that must be weighed carefully. This patient has a full stomach and is at risk for pulmonary aspiration. More importantly, his brief loss of consciousness represents a mild form of traumatic brain injury which can result in impaired cerebral autoregulation and cerebral edema. A hypertensive response to intubation and/or surgical stimulation may elevate intracranial pressure to a degree sufficient to worsen his neurologic status. Finally, some evidence shows that inhaled volatile anesthesia in the setting of concussion promotes brain edema.

2. **Epidural anesthesia:** this would allow for a discrete band of analgesia of the abdominal wall while leaving the sensorium relatively intact. Note that any sedation given to supplement a regional anesthetic technique may result in hypercarbia and increased intracranial pressure.

3. **Peripheral nerve block:** because of the extensive length of the laceration, a large area of the abdominal wall must be blocked. Options include thoracic paravertebral blockade and transversus abdominis plane (TAP) blocks.

4. **Local anesthesia:** not ideal owing to the extensive size of the laceration and the potential for toxicity with large volumes of local anesthetic.

What are the advantages of TAP block in trauma patients?

Advantages include:

- Superior analgesia to placebo
- Avoidance of central neuraxial blockade in patients with established coagulopathy
- Ability to reduce opioid dose and opioid-related side effects
- Improved time to extubation following laparotomy.

You elect to perform bilateral continuous TAP blocks for this patient.

What are the technical considerations for TAP block?

Successful TAP blockade relies on guiding a needle with ultrasound to the plane between the transversus abdominis and internal oblique muscles, and depositing a large volume of local anesthetic to block the intercostal nerves traveling around the side of the trunk (Figure 21.1).

Imaging of the abdominal wall between the costal margin and the iliac crest reveals three muscle layers, separated by hyperechoic fascia: the outermost external oblique (EO), the internal oblique (IO) and the transversus abdominis muscles (TA) (Figure 21.2). Immediately below this last muscle is the transversalis fascia, followed by the peritoneum and the intestines below, which can be visualized moving with peristalsis. The nerves of the abdominal wall are not consistently visible in the TAP.

The distribution of abdominal wall anesthesia following TAP block has not been entirely agreed upon. Most authors agree that reliable blockade of dermatomes L1–T10 can be achieved with usual volumes of local anesthetic. Claims of blockade up to T7 have been made, but these results are not consistently reproducible. This may be related to the choice of technique – some clinicians claim that an injection performed more posteriorly (close to the posterolateral iliac crest) may capture higher-order branches of the T7–L1 nerves in close proximity before they diverge in the anterior abdominal wall. This has not been clarified sufficiently in the literature. Three distinct approaches have been described (subcostal, posterior/triangle of Petit and midaxillary), although superiority has not been shown definitively for any one technique and the most common approach remains the midaxillary, as described below.

Typically this block is performed in the supine position. The iliac crest and costal margin should be palpated and the space between them (usually 5–10 cm) identified as the transducer location. Pediatric patients are almost always induced with general anesthesia prior to the block; this is an option for adults as well.

With the patient supine, the skin is disinfected and the transducer placed on the skin. The three muscle layers should be identified. Sliding the transducer slightly cephalad or caudad will make the muscles appear to move, aiding in identifying them. Once oriented, a skin wheal is then made 2–3 cm medial to the medial aspect of the transducer, and the needle

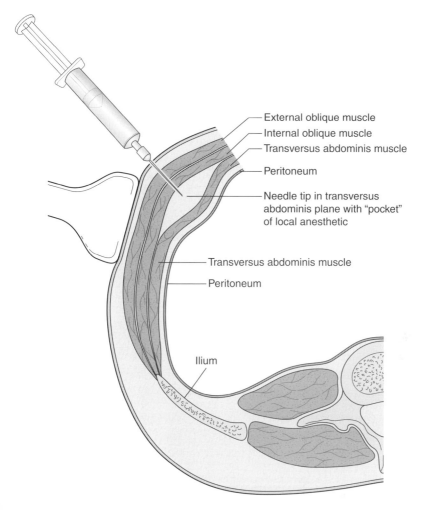

- External oblique muscle
- Internal oblique muscle
- Transversus abdominis muscle
- Peritoneum
- Needle tip in transversus abdominis plane with "pocket" of local anesthetic
- Transversus abdominis muscle
- Peritoneum
- Ilium

Figure 21.1 Transverse section of the abdominal wall showing the three muscle layers. The TAP block is performed by placing the local anesthetic between the internal oblique and transversus abdominis layers.

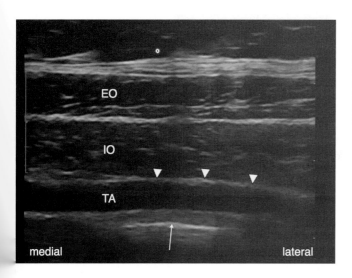

EO

IO

TA

medial   lateral

Figure 21.2 Sonoanatomy relevant to the TAP block. Arrowheads correspond to the target plane between the internal oblique (IO) and transversus abdominis (TA) muscles. Note the peritoneum (arrow) immediately deep to the transversalis fascia. EO, External oblique.

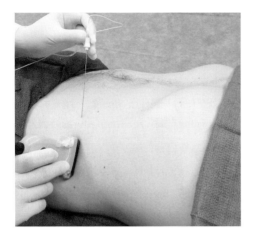

Figure 21.3 Transducer and needle position for ultrasound-guided TAP block. A relatively long needle (100 mm) is used to keep the needle path shallow with respect to the surface of the transducer, thereby increasing the likelihood of visualization.

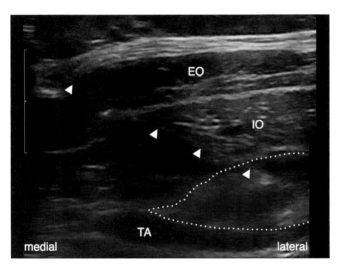

Figure 21.4 Muscle layers of the abdominal wall showing a needle (arrowheads) extending to the transversus abdominis plane. Local anesthetic has been injected, depressing the transversus abdominis muscle (TA) and creating an elongated pocket of injectate (dotted section) that will anesthetize the nerves. EO, External oblique; IO, internal oblique.

inserted in-plane in a medial-to-lateral orientation (Figure 21.3). The needle is guided through the subcutaneous tissue, external oblique muscle and internal oblique muscle. A "pop" may be seen and felt as the needletip enters the plane between the two muscles. After gentle aspiration, 1–2 ml of local anesthetic is injected to verify needletip location. When injection of the local anesthetic appears to be intramuscular, the needle is advanced carefully another 1–2 mm and another bolus administered. This is repeated until spread in the correct plane is achieved (Figure 21.4).

In an adult patient, 20 ml of local anesthetic per side is usually sufficient for successful blockade. In children, a volume of 0.4 ml/kg per side is adequate for effective analgesia when using ultrasound guidance.

How well do TAP blocks work?

The established literature on TAP blocks is somewhat contradictory. In a recent systematic review, Abdallah and colleagues (2012) examined 18 randomized controlled studies that have been published on the topic and came to the following conclusions.

- TAP blocks are safe. No trial reported any block-related complications.
- TAP blocks provide some analgesic benefit for a variety of surgical procedures, but the success depends on many factors, such as the needle insertion site and the relative contribution of visceral versus abdominal wall pain. Examples of procedures that seem to benefit are colorectal surgery, appendectomy (open or laparoscopic) and laparoscopic cholecystectomy.
- Three general techniques for where the block is performed have been described: at the midaxillary line, just above the iliac crest in the so-called triangle of Petit and in the subcostal area. There may be a trend towards improved success when the triangle of Petit approach is used.
- There does not seem to be an association between local anesthetic concentration and block success, and concentrations as low as 0.2% ropivacaine appear to be adequate.
- Finally, TAP block is a compartmental field block, requiring a sufficient volume of local anesthetic (at least 15–20 ml per side) to effect adequate dermatomal spread.

The procedure is completed uneventfully and the wound is closed primarily. The TAP catheters are connected to infusion pumps set to deliver 8 ml/h each or 0.2% ropivacaine. The next day the patient is evaluated by an orthopedic surgeon and is found to have a ruptured anterior cruciate ligament (ACL) of his left knee. A decision is made to discharge the patient home and schedule him for outpatient arthroscopic ACL reconstruction in 3 weeks' time.

The patient desires as little pain as possible postoperatively. What is your analgesic plan for the ACL reconstruction?

Reconstruction of the ACL is a moderately painful procedure. In many centers it is performed as an outpatient procedure, making effective pain control more challenging. The use of continuous catheter techniques in this population can be very effective, particularly in those patients who are at risk for opioid-related side effects. ACL reconstruction is typically performed under combined general anesthesia with laryngeal mask airway and some combination of peripheral nerve blocks. The blocks are always put in after induction of general anesthesia but before surgery, to reduce the requirement for intraoperative opioids and to improve recovery.

The choice of which single-injection and continuous blocks to perform depends largely on the extent of the procedure. All patients in our practice receive a femoral nerve block. If the surgeon plans on harvesting hamstring tendon autograft, a sciatic nerve block should be considered as an adjunct. Finally, despite femoral and sciatic blockade, many patients still experience pain in the posteromedial aspect of the knee, an area that is innervated by articular branches of the obturator nerve. For this reason, an obturator block is usually performed at the time of femoral blockade.

General anesthesia is induced and the femoral catheter is successfully placed. The surgeon is planning on using cadaveric allograft tendon so sciatic nerve block is not performed. You elect to perform an obturator block before the surgery commences.

What are the technical aspects of performing an ultrasound-guided obturator block?

Obturator nerve block is easily performed before or after femoral nerve block. The patient is kept in the same position (supine) and access to the block area can be made easier by externally rotating the thigh and abducting it slightly. The same linear transducer is slid medially several centimeters from where the femoral vessels are usually imaged (Figure 21.5). At this point, the femoral vein should just have disappeared from the lateral aspect of the image. Four muscles should be evident on the ultrasound image: pectineus, adductor longus, adductor brevis and adductor magnus (Figure 21.6). Situated in the planes between adductor longus, brevis and pectineus is the anterior branch of the obturator nerve. Similarly, the posterior branch lies in the fascial plane between adductor brevis and magnus.

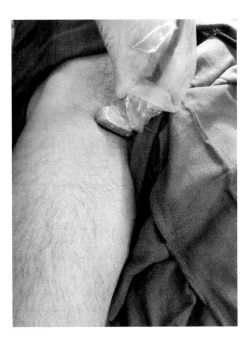

Figure 21.5 Transducer position for ultrasound-guided obturator nerve block. The thigh is slightly externally rotated and abducted.

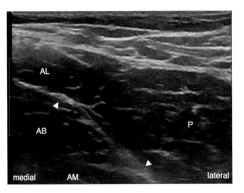

Figure 21.6 Sonoanatomy relevant to the ultrasound-guided obturator nerve block. Arrowheads correspond to the anterior and posterior branches of the obturator nerve. The anterior branch is located superficially between adductor longus (AL) and brevis (AB), while the posterior branch can be found in the plane separating adductor brevis, adductor magnus (AM) and pectineus (P).

The goal of the block is to put 5–10 ml of local anesthetic in the intermuscular planes for each nerve. Both nerves supply motor innervation to the adductor group, but only the posterior branch supplies articular branches to the knee. As such, we typically only block the posterior branch for ACL surgery. The anterior branch carries articular fibers to the hip joint, but they depart the main nerve proximal to this level and a lumbar plexus block is required to block those twigs effectively.

A 10-cm block needle can be advanced in-plane from the medial side, taking care not to puncture the femoral vein, or out-of-plane. Both approaches are easy and both are associated with excellent success rates. Nerve stimulation is a helpful confirmatory tool; needletip location within the adductor muscle will result in a mild diffuse twitch but, when stimulating either branch of the nerve, a brisk adduction response of the thigh is observed.

References and further reading

Abdallah, F. W., Chan, V. W., Brull, R. (2012). Transversus abdominis plane block: a systematic review. *Regional Anesthesia and Pain Medicine*, 37, 193–209.

Allcock, E., Spencer, E., Frazer, R., Applegate, G., Buckenmaier, C., 3rd. (2010). Continuous transversus abdominis plane (TAP) block catheters in a combat surgical environment. *Pain Medicine (Malden, Mass.)*, 11, 1426–9.

Hebbard, P. D., Barrington, M. J., Vasey, C. (2010). Ultrasound-guided continuous oblique subcostal transversus abdominis plane blockade: description of anatomy and clinical technique. *Regional Anesthesia and Pain Medicine*, 35, 436–41.

Lee, T. H. W., Barrington, M. J., Tran, T. M. N., Wong, D., Hebbard, P. D. (2010). Comparison of extent of sensory block following posterior and subcostal approaches to ultrasound-guided transversus abdominis plane block. *Anaesthesia and Intensive Care*, 38, 452–60.

Niraj, G., Kelkar, A., Jeyapalan, I. et al. (2011). Comparison of analgesic efficacy of subcostal transversus abdominis plane blocks with epidural analgesia following upper abdominal surgery. *Anaesthesia*, 66, 465–71.

Sakura, S., Hara, K., Ota, J., Tadenuma, S. (2010). Ultrasound-guided peripheral nerve blocks for anterior cruciate ligament reconstruction: effect of obturator nerve block during and after surgery. *Journal of Anesthesia*, 24, 411–17.

Sinha, S. K., Abrams, J. H., Houle, T. T., Weller, R. S. (2009). Ultrasound-guided obturator nerve block: an interfascial injection approach without nerve stimulation. *Regional Anesthesia and Pain Medicine*, 34, 261–4.

Index